THE Low-FODMAP Diet Cookbook 2024

Delicious, Gut-Friendly Low-FODMAP Recipes to Reduce IBS, Manage Digestive Disorders and Enjoy Every Meal with 28-Day Meal Plan

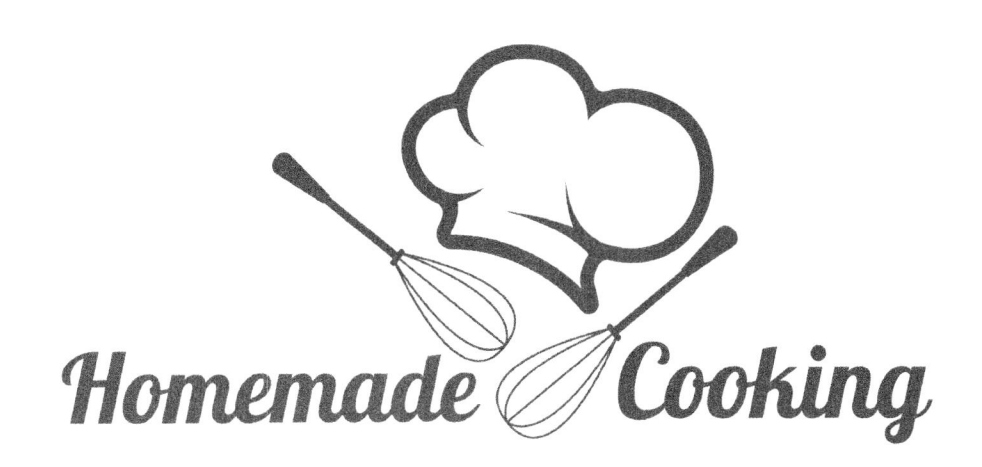

Homemade Cooking

Sandra J. Hampton

Copyright © 2024 by Sandra J. Hampton

All rights reserved.

This recipe book and its contents are protected by copyright law. The recipes, photographs, and words within these pages are the fruits of our passion for cooking. We kindly ask that you respect our creative efforts by refraining from reproducing, storing, or sharing any part of this book without our prior written consent.

Cooking is an art, and like any art form, it carries inherent risks. While we've strived to provide safe and accurate recipes, results may vary. We assume no liability for accidents, injuries, or allergies that may occur during cooking. Exercise caution, adhere to food safety guidelines, and consult experts when needed.

Thank you for choosing Sandra J. Hampton's The Low-FODMAP Diet Cookbook 2024. Your support means the world to us, and we hope our recipes bring warmth and flavor to your culinary journey. By using this book, you agree to respect our copyright terms and understand our disclaimer.

Happy cooking

Sincerely,

Sandra J. Hampton

CONTENTS

INTRODUCTION 7
IBS, What, Why and How to 8
Gradually Understanding Low-FODMAP Diet 9
Common Low-FODMAP and High-FODMAP Foods 10
Questions you may care about 10

28-Day Meal Plan 12

Breakfast & Brunch Recipes 14
Scrambled Tofu 15
Cucumber Salad 15
Jubilant Muesli Mix 15
Dressed-up Eggs 15
Savory Muffins 16
Rhubarb Ginger Granola Bowl 16
Basil Vinaigrette Salad Dressing 16
Ginger-berry Rice Milk Smoothie 16
Easy Breakfast Sausage 17
Blueberry, Lime, And Coconut Smoothie 17
Chia Seed Carrot Cake Pudding 17
Pb&j Smoothie 17
Strawberry Smoothie 17
Melon And Yogurt Parfait 18
Crêpes With Cheese Sauce 18
Basil Omelet With Smashed Tomato 18
Cinnamon Spice Granola 19
Banana Toast 19
Breakfast Tortillas 19
Banana Oatcakes 19
Egg Wraps 20
Amaranth Breakfast 20
Crispy Noodle Cakes With Chili Sauce 20
Coconut Cacao Hazelnut Smoothie Bowl 21
Bacon And Zucchini Crustless Quiche 21
High-fiber Muffins With Zucchini And Sunflower Seeds 21
Blueberry Lime Smoothie 21
Crunchy Granola 22
Carrot Cake Porridge 22
Chicken Liver Pâté With Pepper And Sage 22
Breakfast Ratatouille With Poached Eggs 22
Quinoa Porridge 23
Chili-cheese Muffins 23
Quinoa Breakfast Bowl With Basil "hollandaise" Sauce 23
Pesto Noodles 24
Green Dragon Smoothie Bowl 24
Fried Eggs With Potato Hash 24

Soups, Salads And Sides Recipes. 25
Rice Paper "spring Rolls" With Satay Sauce 26
Lemony Grilled Zucchini With Feta And Pine Nuts.26
Caramelized Squash Salad With Sun-dried Tomatoes And Basil 26
Roasted Squash And Chestnut Soup 26
Chicken And Dumplings Soup 27
Roasted Sweet Potato Salad With Spiced Lamb And Spinach 27
Orange-maple Glazed Carrots 28
Easy Onion- And Garlic-free Chicken Stock 28
Coconut Rice 28
Roasted Potato Wedges 28
Mussels In Chili, Bacon, And Tomato Broth 28
Quinoa With Cherry Tomatoes, Olives, And Radishes 29
Sesame Rice Noodles 29
Chive Dip 29
Turkey-ginger Soup 29
Classic Coleslaw 30
Blue Cheese And Arugula Salad With Red Wine Dressing 30
Bacon Mashed Potatoes 30
Prosciutto Di Parma Salad 30
Potato Leek Soup 31
Abundantly Happy Kale Salad 31
Beetroot Dip 31

Veggie Dip 31
Quinoa With Swiss Chard 32
Butter Lettuce Salad With Poached Egg And Bacon 32
Roasted Vegetable Soup 32
Zucchini Ribbon Salad With Goat Cheese, Pine Nuts, And Pomegranate 32
Roast Vegetables 33
Creamy Seafood Soup 33
Fennel Pomegranate Salad 33
Kale And Red Bell Pepper Salad 34
Pesto Ham Sandwich 34
Hearty Lamb Shank And Vegetable Soup 34
Kale Sesame Salad With Tamari-ginger Dressing 34
Philly Steak Sandwich 35
Mom's Chicken Salad 35
Roman Egg Drop Soup 35

Fish And Seafood Recipes 36

Summery Fish Stew 37
Coconut Shrimp 37
Atlantic Cod With Basil Walnut Sauce 37
Rita's Linguine With Clam Sauce 37
Shrimp And Cheese Casserole 38
Creamy Halibut 38
Shrimp Puttanesca With Linguine 38
Cornmeal-crusted Tilapia 38
Salmon Noodle Casserole 39
Light Tuna Casserole 39
Salmon Cakes With Fresh Dill Sauce 40
Grilled Cod With Fresh Basil 40
Seafood Risotto 40
Mediterranean Flaky Fish With Vegetables 40
Tilapia Piccata 41
Basic Baked Scallops 41
Grilled Halibut With Lemony Pesto 41
Baked Moroccan-style Halibut 42
Poached Salmon With Tarragon Sauce 42
Cedar Planked Salmon 42
Glazed Salmon 42
Coconut-crusted Fish With Pineapple Relish 43
Grilled Swordfish With Pineapple Salsa 43
Sole Meunière 43
Citrusy Swordfish Skewers 43
Shrimp With Cherry Tomatoes 44
Salmon With Herbs 44
Feta Crab Cakes 44

Maple-glazed Salmon 45
Fish And Chips 45

Vegetarian And Vegan Recipes 46

Tempeh Tacos 47
Tofu And Red Bell Pepper Quinoa 47
Vegan Noodles With Gingered Coconut Sauce 47
Roasted-veggie Gyros With Tzatziki Sauce 48
Stuffed Zucchini Boats 48
Cheese Strata 48
Mac 'n' Cheeze 49
Kale-pesto Soba Noodles 49
Curried Squash Soup With Coconut Milk 49
Polenta With Roasted Vegetables And Spicy Tomato Sauce 50
Coconut-curry Tofu With Vegetables 50
Zucchini Pizza Bites 50
Vegetable Stir-fry 51
Pasta With Tomato And Lentil Sauce 51
Vegan Pad Thai 51
Collard Green Wraps With Thai Peanut Dressing 51
Pineapple Fried Rice 52
Tempeh Enchiladas With Red Chili Sauce 52
Eggplant And Chickpea Curry 52
Zucchini Pasta Alla Puttanesca 53
Lemon And Mozzarella Polenta Pizza 53
Summer Vegetable Pasta 53
Vegetable And Rice Noodle Bowl 54
Baked Tofu Báhn Mì Lettuce Wrap 54
Pasta With Pesto Sauce 54
Tempeh Lettuce Wraps 55
Mediterranean Noodles 55
Mixed Grains, Seeds, And Vegetable Bowl 55
Turmeric Rice With Cranberries 55
Vegan Potato Salad, Cypriot-style 56
Baked Tofu And Vegetables 56
Vegetable Fried Rice 56
Watercress Zucchini Soup 57
Latin Quinoa-stuffed Peppers 57
Tofu Burger Patties 57
Moroccan-spiced Lentil And Quinoa Stew 58
Chipotle Tofu And Sweet Potato Tacos With Avocado Salsa 58

Meat Recipes ... 59

- Grilled Chicken Parmigiana ... 60
- Mild Lamb Curry ... 60
- Chili-rubbed Pork Chops With Raspberry Sauce ... 60
- Chinese Chicken ... 61
- Orange-ginger Salmon ... 61
- Creamy Smoked Salmon Pasta ... 61
- Spicy Pulled Pork ... 62
- Baked Chicken And Mozzarella Croquettes ... 62
- Lemon Thyme Chicken ... 62
- Pork And Fennel Meatballs ... 63
- Pan-fried Chicken With Brown Butter–sage Sauce .. 63
- Garden Veggie Dip Burgers ... 63
- Chicken Tenders ... 63
- Chicken Parmigiana ... 64
- Stuffed Rolled Roast Beef With Popovers And Gravy 64
- Chicken Pockets ... 65
- Lamb And Vegetable Pilaf ... 65
- Chicken And Rice With Peanut Sauce ... 66
- Pecan-crusted Maple-mustard Salmon ... 66
- Pumpkin Maple Roast Chicken ... 66
- Chimichurri Chicken Drumsticks ... 66
- Crispy Baked Chicken With Gravy ... 67
- Thai Sweet Chili Broiled Salmon ... 67
- Spinach And Feta-stuffed Chicken Breast ... 67
- Italian-herbed Chicken Meatballs In Broth ... 68
- Turkey Dijon ... 68
- Easy Pan Chicken ... 68
- Stuffed Peppers With Ground Turkey ... 69
- Dijon-roasted Pork Tenderloin ... 69
- Asian-style Pork Meatballs ... 69
- Fish With Thai Red Curry Sauce ... 70
- Beef Stir-fry With Chinese Broccoli And Green Beans 70
- Soy-infused Roast Chicken ... 70
- Snapper With Tropical Salsa ... 71
- Polenta-crusted Chicken ... 71
- Quick Meatloaf Patties ... 71
- Lemon-pepper Shrimp ... 71

Sauces, Dressings, And Condiments Recipes ... 72

- Luscious Hot Fudge Sauce ... 73
- Low-fodmap Poultry Broth Or Meat Broth ... 73
- Pumpkin Maple Glaze ... 73
- Tomato Paste ... 73
- Tahini Dressing ... 74
- Thai Red Curry Paste ... 74
- Basic Mayonnaise ... 74
- Low-fodmap Worcestershire Sauce ... 74
- Fiesta Salsa ... 75
- Ginger Sesame Salad Dressing ... 75
- Garlic-infused Oil ... 75
- Sun-dried Tomato Pesto ... 75
- Egg-free Caesar Dressing ... 75
- Raspberry Sauce ... 76
- Garlic Oil ... 76
- Low-fodmap Mayonnaise ... 76
- Sweet Chili Garlic Sauce ... 76
- Olive Tapenade ... 76
- Autumn's Glaze ... 77
- Low-fodmap Vegetable Broth ... 77
- Basil Sauce ... 77
- Dill Dipping Sauce ... 77
- Macadamia Spinach Pesto ... 77
- Tangy Lemon Curd ... 78
- Maple Dressing ... 78
- Caesar Salad Dressing ... 78
- Aioli ... 78
- Artisanal Ketchup ... 78
- Basil "hollandaise" Sauce ... 79
- Low-fodmap Spicy Ketchup ... 79
- Homemade Mayonnaise ... 79
- Sweet Barbecue Sauce ... 79
- Steakhouse Rub ... 80
- Strawberry Chia Seed Jam ... 80
- Chimichurri Sauce ... 80
- Italian Basil Vinaigrette ... 80
- Salsa Verde ... 80

Snacks & Desserts Recipes 81

Cinnamon And Chestnut Flan 82
Easy Trail Mix 82
Caramelized Upside-down Banana Cake 82
Parmesan Potato Wedges 83
Lemon Coconut Cupcakes 83
Crispy Gluten-free Chocolate Chip Cookies 83
Sweet And Savory Popcorn 84
Berry Crumble 84
Peanut Butter Cookies 84
Maple-spiced Walnuts 84
Rich White Chocolate Cake 85
Salted Caramel Pumpkin Seeds 85
Strawberry Ice Cream 85
Herbed Rice Fritters With Parmesan Cheese 86
Chocolate Peanut Butter Cups 86
Pineapple Salsa 86
Fluffy Pancakes 86
Lemon Tartlets 87
Dark Chocolate–macadamia Nut Brownies 87
Baked Oat Cup 87
Rhubarb Custard Cup 88
Chocolate Lava Cakes 88
Banana Birthday Cake With Lemon Icing 88
Lemon Tart 89
Amaretti 89
Chia Pudding 89
Pineapple Sorbet 90
Vietnamese Shrimp-and-herb Spring Rolls 90
Peanut Butter And Sesame Cookies 90
Herbed Polenta "fries" 91
Chocolate Peanut Butter Energy Bites 91
No-bake Coconut Cookie Bars 91
Caramel Nut Bars 91
Chocolate-mint Bars 92
Chocolate Truffles 92
Brownie Cupcakes With Vanilla Icing 93
Citrus Rice Tart With Raspberry Sauce 93

Shopping List 95

Appendix A : Measurement Conversions 96

Appendix B : Recipes Index 98

INTRODUCTION

Sandra J. Hampton is a seasoned dietitian, nutritionist, and culinary enthusiast with a passion for creating delicious, gut-friendly recipes. With over two decades of experience in the field of nutrition and dietetics, she has become a trusted expert in helping individuals manage their digestive health and improve their overall well-being.

Sandra's journey towards writing her highly acclaimed "Low-FODMAP Cookbook" began with a deep empathy for those suffering from Irritable Bowel Syndrome (IBS) and related gastrointestinal disorders. Her work as a clinical dietitian exposed her to countless patients struggling to find relief from the daily challenges of digestive discomfort. This experience ignited her determination to provide practical solutions through the power of food.

Drawing from her extensive education in nutrition, including a Master's degree in Clinical Nutrition, Sandra embarked on a meticulous research process. She delved into the intricate world of FODMAPs (Fermentable Oligosaccharides, Disaccharides, Monosaccharides, and Polyols), gaining a profound understanding of their impact on gut health and how certain dietary modifications can alleviate symptoms.

Sandra's background in the culinary arts was an invaluable asset in developing her cookbook. With a creative flair in the kitchen and a knack for transforming everyday ingredients into mouthwatering dishes, she set out to create a collection of recipes that would prove that a low-FODMAP diet could be both nutritious and delightful.

Her writing process involved hours of recipe testing, experimenting with various combinations of ingredients, and refining her culinary techniques to ensure that each dish not only met the strict dietary requirements but also tantalized the taste buds. Her dedication to producing a cookbook that catered to the diverse palates of her readers shines through in every carefully crafted recipe.

Sandra's "Low-FODMAP Cookbook" is the culmination of her expertise, passion, and commitment to improving the lives of individuals managing digestive issues. With this book, she offers a treasure trove of flavorful recipes, practical tips, and expert guidance to help readers navigate the challenges of a low-FODMAP diet with ease and enjoyment.

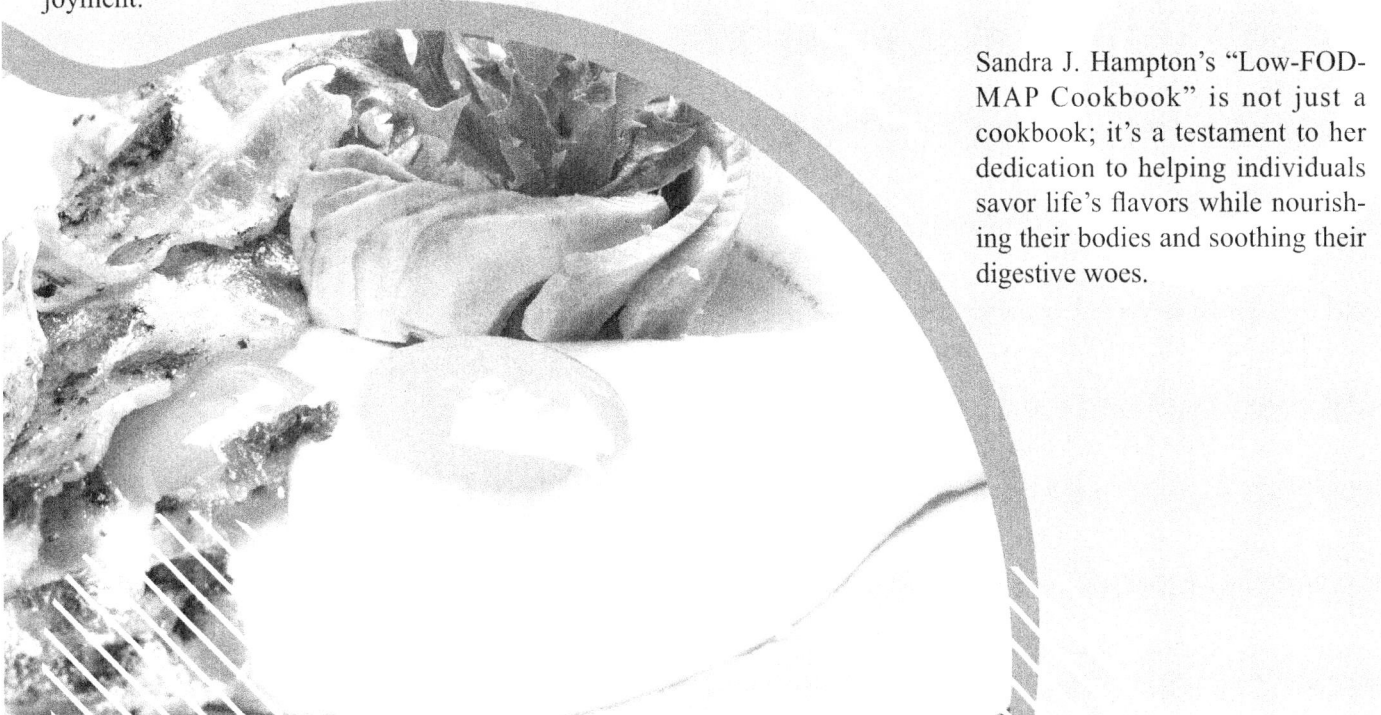

Sandra J. Hampton's "Low-FODMAP Cookbook" is not just a cookbook; it's a testament to her dedication to helping individuals savor life's flavors while nourishing their bodies and soothing their digestive woes.

IBS, What, Why and How to

What

Irritable Bowel Syndrome (IBS) is a common gastrointestinal disorder that affects the large intestine (colon) and often causes a range of digestive symptoms. It is considered a functional gastrointestinal disorder, which means that it doesn't have a known structural or biochemical cause. Instead, IBS is characterized by a cluster of symptoms, which can vary from person to person.

Why

Irritable Bowel Syndrome (IBS) occurs due to a combination of factors, including abnormal gut motility, heightened sensitivity of the intestines, altered gut microbiome, dietary triggers, psychological stressors, and potential genetic predispositions. This multifactorial disorder leads to a range of gastrointestinal symptoms such as abdominal pain, altered bowel habits, bloating, and discomfort. While the exact cause remains unclear, it is often diagnosed after ruling out other gastrointestinal conditions.

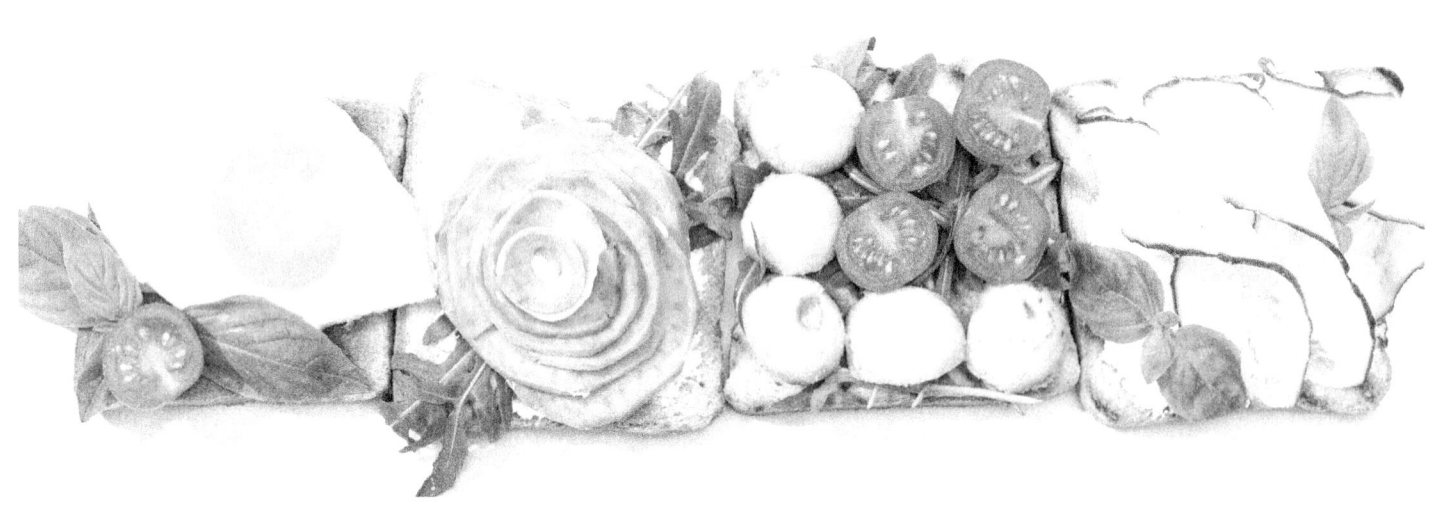

How to

1. Consult a Healthcare Provider:

If you suspect you have IBS, it's essential to seek a healthcare provider's diagnosis and guidance. They can rule out other conditions and tailor a treatment plan to your specific symptoms.

2. Dietary Modifications:

Identify Trigger Foods: Keep a food diary to track what you eat and how it affects your symptoms. Common triggers include FODMAPs, dairy, caffeine, and high-fat foods.

Low-FODMAP Diet: Some individuals find relief by following a low-FODMAP diet under the guidance of a registered dietitian.

Balanced Diet: Aim for a well-balanced diet with plenty of fiber from fruits, vegetables, and whole grains.

Hydration: Drink enough water to prevent dehydration and aid digestion.

3. Stress Management:

Practice stress reduction techniques such as deep breathing, meditation, yoga, or mindfulness.

Regular exercise can help reduce stress and improve bowel function.

4. Lifestyle Changes:

Get regular, adequate sleep.

Avoid smoking and excessive alcohol consumption.

Limit or avoid caffeine intake.

Eat smaller, more frequent meals to prevent overloading your digestive system.

Avoid eating large meals close to bedtime.

Gradually Understanding Low-FODMAP Diet

The Low-FODMAP Diet is a dietary approach designed to manage and alleviate symptoms in individuals with Irritable Bowel Syndrome (IBS) and certain other gastrointestinal conditions. FODMAPs are short-chain carbohydrates that are poorly absorbed in the small intestine and can ferment in the colon, leading to gas, bloating, abdominal pain, and diarrhea in sensitive individuals. The acronym "FODMAP" stands for Fermentable Oligosaccharides, Disaccharides, Monosaccharides, and Polyols.

FODMAP Categories:

Oligosaccharides: This category includes fructans (found in wheat, onions, and garlic) and galacto-oligosaccharides (found in legumes).

Disaccharides: Lactose, a disaccharide found in dairy products, is a common trigger for many with lactose intolerance.

Monosaccharides: Fructose, both naturally occurring in some fruits and added as high-fructose corn syrup, can be problematic for some individuals.

Polyols: These are sugar alcohols like sorbitol and mannitol, often found in certain fruits (e.g., apples, pears) and artificial sweeteners.

Elimination Phase: The Low-FODMAP Diet typically begins with an elimination phase during which high-FODMAP foods are removed from the diet for a specified period (usually 2-6 weeks) to alleviate symptoms.

Reintroduction Phase: After the elimination phase, individual FODMAP groups are systematically reintroduced one at a time to identify specific triggers and determine tolerance levels. This phase helps create a more personalized and sustainable long-term diet.

Potential Benefits: For many individuals with IBS, the Low-FODMAP Diet can lead to a significant reduction in symptoms, including reduced bloating, gas, diarrhea, and abdominal pain.

Long-Term Diet: The goal is not to follow a strict low-FODMAP diet indefinitely but to identify and manage specific triggers, allowing for a more balanced and varied diet.

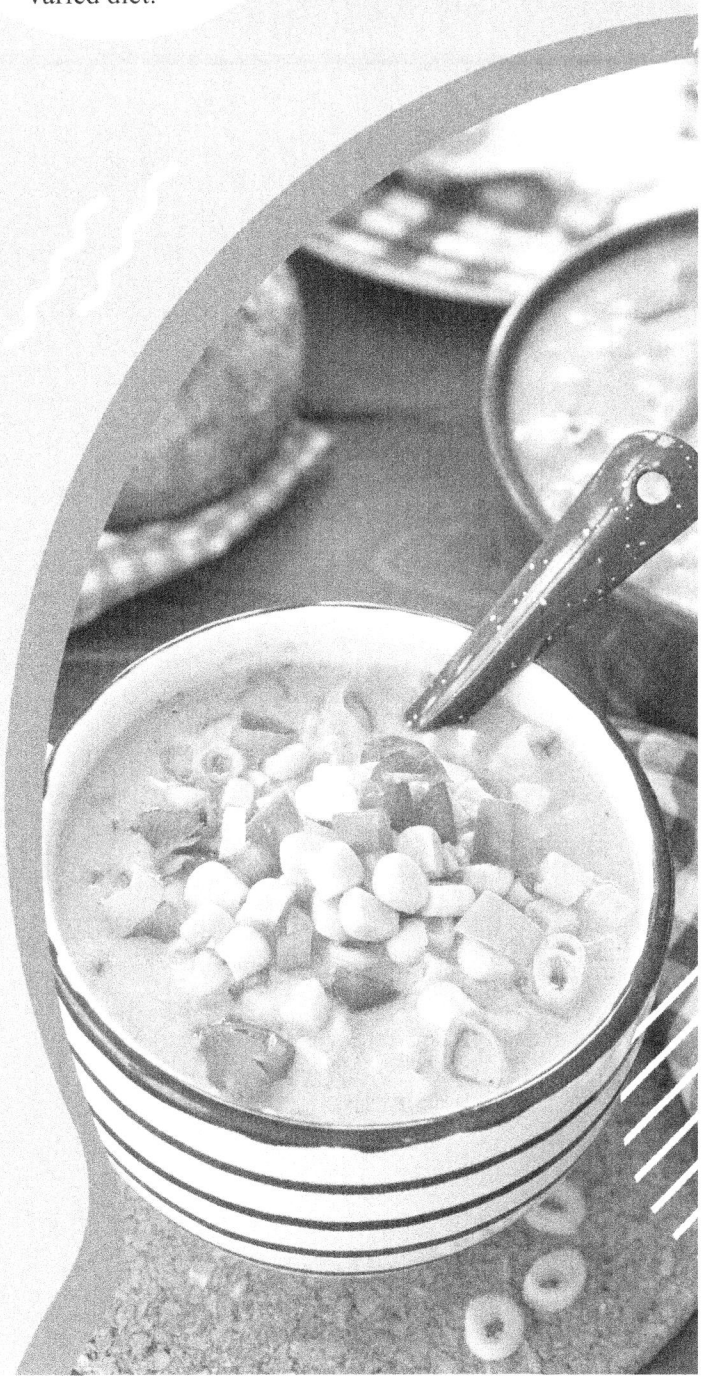

Common Low-FODMAP and High-FODMAP Foods

	Low-FODMAP Foods	High-FODMAP Foods
Fruits	Bananas, Blueberries, Grapes, Kiwi, Oranges, Pineapple	Apples, Cherries, Watermelon, Mango, Pears, Plums
Vegetables	Carrots, Cucumbers, Lettuce, Zucchini, Spinach, Bell peppers	Onions, Garlic, Cauliflower, Mushrooms, Asparagus, Broccoli
Grains	Rice (white and brown), Oats (gluten-free), Quinoa, Polenta, Corn	Wheat-based products (bread, pasta), Barley, Rye, Wheat bran, Bulgur
Proteins	Chicken, Turkey, Fish (salmon, trout, cod), Eggs, Firm tofu	Legumes (beans, lentils, chickpeas), Tofu, Processed meats (sausages, bacon), Cashews, Pistachios
Dairy	Lactose-free milk, Hard cheeses (cheddar, Swiss), Greek yogurt (low-lactose), Butter (lactose-free), Dairy-free alternatives (almond, soy)	Regular cow's milk, Soft cheeses (ricotta, cottage cheese), Ice cream, Cream cheese, Evaporated milk
Sweeteners	Maple syrup, Stevia, Sugar (table sugar), Brown sugar (in moderation), Artificial sweeteners (aspartame)	High-fructose corn syrup, Honey, Agave nectar, Sorbitol, Xylitol

Questions you may care about

WHAT DIETARY CHANGES CAN HELP MANAGE IBS SYMPTOMS?

Dietary modifications can play a significant role in managing IBS. Many individuals find relief by following a low-FODMAP diet, which reduces the consumption of specific fermentable carbohydrates. Other dietary strategies may include avoiding trigger foods, increasing fiber intake, and staying hydrated.

CAN STRESS AND ANXIETY EXACERBATE IBS SYMPTOMS?

Yes, stress and anxiety can trigger or worsen IBS symptoms in many individuals. Stress management techniques, relaxation exercises, and, in some cases, therapy can be beneficial in reducing symptom severity.

HOW IS THE LOW-FODMAP DIET IMPLEMENTED?

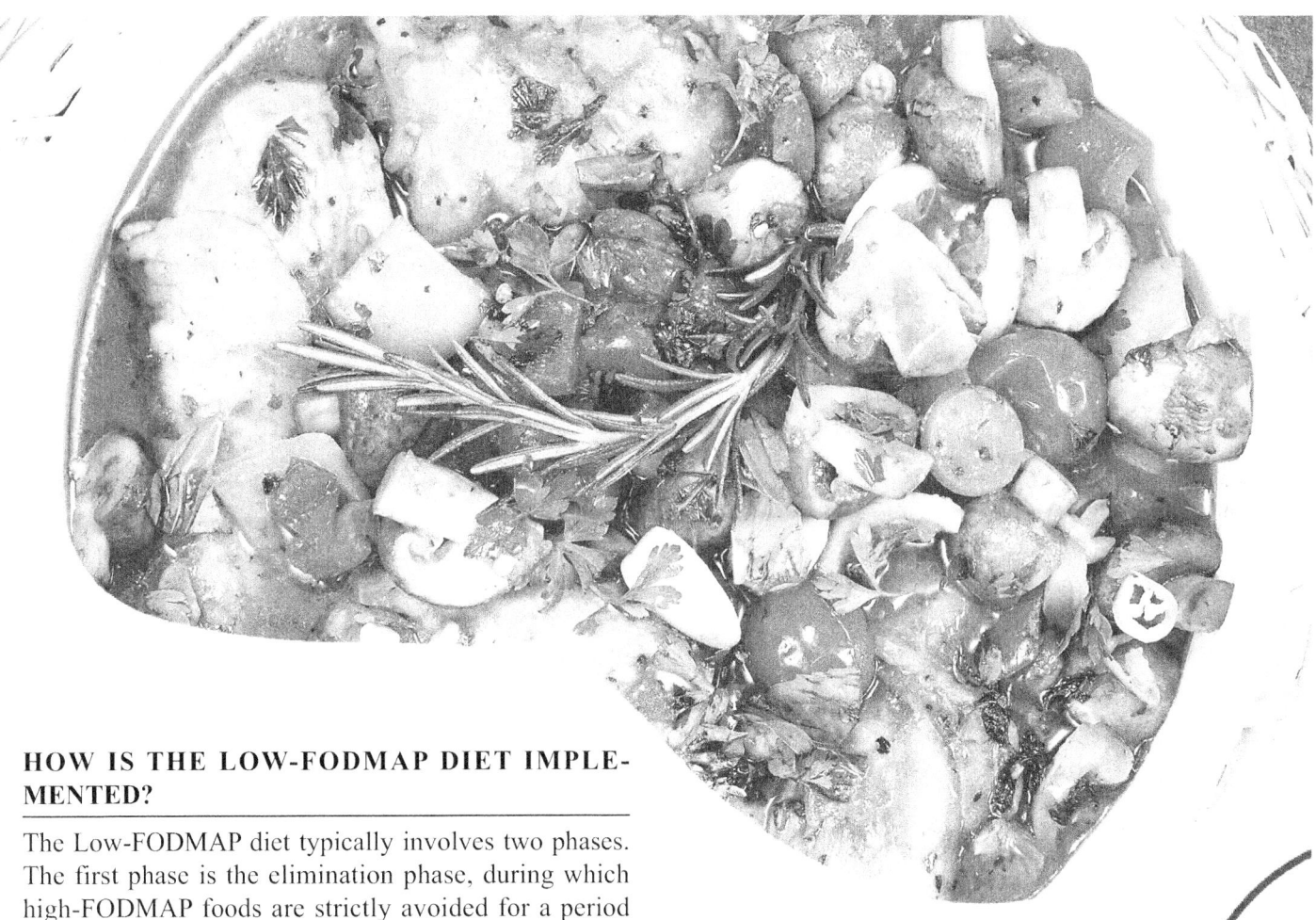

The Low-FODMAP diet typically involves two phases. The first phase is the elimination phase, during which high-FODMAP foods are strictly avoided for a period of 2-6 weeks. The second phase is the reintroduction phase, in which specific FODMAP-containing foods are gradually reintroduced to determine which ones trigger symptoms.

IS THE LOW-FODMAP DIET A LONG-TERM SOLUTION?

The Low-FODMAP diet is typically not intended to be a long-term solution. After completing the elimination and reintroduction phases, individuals can identify their specific trigger foods and develop a personalized dietary plan. Many people find that they can enjoy a varied diet with fewer restrictions once they understand their FODMAP triggers.

SHOULD I UNDERTAKE THE LOW-FODMAP DIET ON MY OWN?

It is highly recommended to undertake the Low-FODMAP diet under the guidance of a registered dietitian or healthcare professional who specializes in gastrointestinal disorders. They can provide personalized guidance, ensure nutritional balance, and help monitor your progress.

CAN I STILL ENJOY A BALANCED DIET ON THE LOW-FODMAP DIET?

Yes, it is possible to maintain a balanced diet on the Low-FODMAP diet by selecting appropriate low-FODMAP foods from all food groups. A dietitian can help you create a well-balanced meal plan to meet your nutritional needs.

CAN THE LOW-FODMAP DIET COMPLETELY ELIMINATE IBS SYMPTOMS?

The Low-FODMAP diet can significantly reduce or even eliminate IBS symptoms for many individuals. However, its effectiveness varies from person to person. It's essential to work closely with a healthcare professional to determine the most suitable dietary approach and to address other factors that may contribute to IBS symptoms, such as stress and anxiety.

28-Day Meal Plan

DAY	BREAKFAST	LUNCH	DINNER
1	Cucumber Salad 15	Scrambled Tofu 15	Summery Fish Stew 37
2	Jubilant Muesli Mix 15	Carrot Cake Porridge 22	Coconut Shrimp 37
3	Savory Muffins 16	Chicken Liver Pâté With Pepper And Sage 22	Atlantic Cod With Basil Walnut Sauce 37
4	Rhubarb Ginger Granola Bowl 16	Quinoa Porridge 23	Rita's Linguine With Clam Sauce 37
5	Basil Vinaigrette Salad Dressing 16	Chili-cheese Muffins 23	Shrimp And Cheese Casserole 38
6	Dressed-up Eggs 15	Pesto Noodles 24	Creamy Halibut 38
7	Ginger-berry Rice Milk Smoothie 16	Fried Eggs With Potato Hash 24	Shrimp Puttanesca With Linguine 38
8	Easy Breakfast Sausage 17	Green Dragon Smoothie Bowl 24	Cornmeal-crusted Tilapia 38
9	Blueberry, Lime, And Coconut Smoothie 17	Rice Paper "spring Rolls" With Satay Sauce 26	Salmon Noodle Casserole 40
10	Chia Seed Carrot Cake Pudding 17	Lemony Grilled Zucchini With Feta And Pine Nuts 26	Light Tuna Casserole 39
11	Pb&j Smoothie 17	Caramelized Squash Salad With Sun-dried Tomatoes And Basil 26	Salmon Cakes With Fresh Dill Sauce 40
12	Strawberry Smoothie 17	Roasted Squash And Chestnut Soup 26	Grilled Cod With Fresh Basil 40
13	Melon And Yogurt Parfait 18	Chicken And Dumplings Soup 27	Seafood Risotto 40
14	Crêpes With Cheese Sauce 18	Roasted Sweet Potato Salad With Spiced Lamb And Spinach 27	:Mediterranean Flaky Fish With Vegetables 40

Low-FODMAP Diet Cookbook

DAY	BREAKFAST	LUNCH	DINNER
15	Basil Omelet With Smashed Tomato 18	Orange-maple Glazed Carrots 28	Tilapia Piccata 41
16	Cinnamon Spice Granola 19	Easy Onion- And Garlic-free Chicken Stock 28	Basic Baked Scallops 41
17	Banana Toast 19	Coconut Rice 28	Grilled Halibut With Lemony Pesto 41
18	Breakfast Tortillas 19	Roasted Potato Wedges 28	Baked Moroccan-style Halibut 42
19	Banana Oatcakes 19	:Mussels In Chili, Bacon, And Tomato Broth 28	Poached Salmon With Tarragon Sauce 42
20	Egg Wraps 20	Quinoa With Cherry Tomatoes, Olives, And Radishes 29	Cedar Planked Salmon 42
21	Amaranth Breakfast 20	Sesame Rice Noodles 29	Glazed Salmon 42
22	Crispy Noodle Cakes With Chili Sauce 20	Chive Dip 29	Coconut-crusted Fish With Pineapple Relish 43
23	Coconut Cacao Hazelnut Smoothie Bowl 21	Classic Coleslaw 30	Grilled Swordfish With Pineapple Salsa 43
24	Bacon And Zucchini Crustless Quiche 21	Blue Cheese And Arugula Salad With Red Wine Dressing 30	Sole Meunière 43
25	High-fiber Muffins With Zucchini And Sunflower Seeds 21	Bacon Mashed Potatoes 30	Citrusy Swordfish Skewers 43
26	Crunchy Granola 22	Prosciutto Di Parma Salad 30	Shrimp With Cherry Tomatoes 44
27	Blueberry Lime Smoothie 21	Potato Leek Soup 31	Salmon With Herbs 44
28	Breakfast Ratatouille With Poached Eggs 22	Abundantly Happy Kale Salad 31	Feta Crab Cakes 44

Low-FODMAP Diet Cookbook

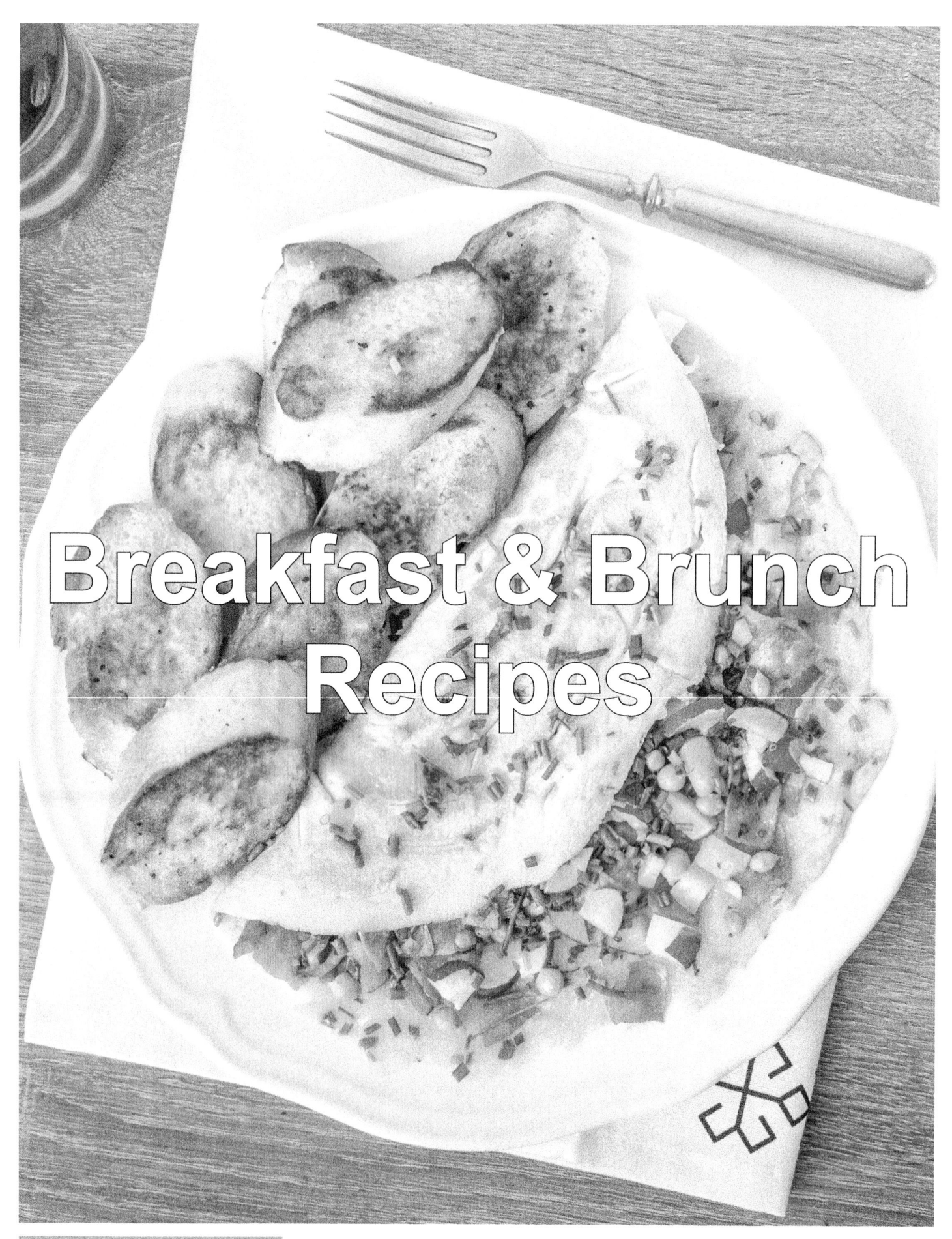

Breakfast & Brunch Recipes

Breakfast & Brunch Recipes

Scrambled Tofu
Servings:1 | Cooking Time: 5 Minutes

Ingredients:
- ½ cup medium-firm tofu
- ¼ cup water
- 1 tbsp soy sauce (gluten-free)
- ¼ tsp turmeric, ground
- ½ cup grated carrot and zucchini
- Oil for greasing the pan
- 1 slice FODMAP-approved bread

Directions:
1. In a bowl, thoroughly mix together the water, soy sauce, and turmeric. Once mixed, add the vegetables and crumble the tofu into the bowl.
2. Place an oil-greased pan onto medium heat and place the mixture in it. Fry the mixture for 5 minutes or until it is golden brown.
3. Serve with a slice of FODMAP-approved toast.

Nutrition Info:
- 82g Calories, 5g Total fat, 0.5g Saturated fat, 4g Carbohydrates, 0.5 g Fiber, 5g Protein, 2g Sodium.

Cucumber Salad
Servings:4 | Cooking Time: -

Ingredients:
- ¾ cup cucumber
- 2 tbsp chives, fresh
- ½ cup Greek yogurt
- ¼ cup white vinegar

Directions:
1. Slice the cucumber thinly and place it into salad bowls along with the yogurt.
2. Chop the chives and mix them into the cucumber along with the vinegar.
3. Refrigerate until you are ready to eat.

Nutrition Info:
- 46.5g Calories, 3g Total fat, 1.75g Saturated fat, 3.5g Carbohydrates, 0.5 g Fiber, 1.75g Protein, 2.25g Sodium.

Jubilant Muesli Mix
Servings:1 | Cooking Time:x

Ingredients:
- 2 teaspoons shredded unsweetened coconut
- 1/2 medium orange, peeled and chopped
- 1/2 tablespoon no-sugar-added dried cranberries
- 1/3 cup lactose-free vanilla yogurt
- 1/3 cup quinoa flakes
- 1/4 cup chia seeds
- 1/8 teaspoon ground nutmeg
- 1/4 teaspoon ground cinnamon
- 1 teaspoon alcohol-free vanilla extract
- 1/8 teaspoon sea salt
- 1/4 cup pumpkin seeds
- 1 tablespoon chopped walnuts
- 1 teaspoon cacao nibs

Directions:
1. Place coconut in a small skillet over medium-high heat. Stir frequently until flakes become golden brown. Remove from heat and set aside. You may also toast coconut in oven: Preheat oven to 350°F. Using a rimmed baking sheet, spread out coconut and toast, tossing occasionally until golden, about 5 minutes. Set aside.
2. In a medium bowl, stir together chopped orange, cranberries, yogurt, quinoa, chia seeds, nutmeg, cinnamon, vanilla extract, and salt. Cover and chill overnight. Just before serving, top with pumpkin seeds, walnuts, cacao, and coconut.

Nutrition Info:
- Calories: 748,Fat: 42g,Protein: 30g,Sodium: 364mg,Carbohydrates: 69.

Dressed-up Eggs
Servings:4 | Cooking Time:x

Ingredients:
- 8 large eggs
- 1 teaspoon unrefined coconut oil, liquefied
- 1 medium tomato, seeded and diced
- 1/4 teaspoon sea salt
- 1/4 teaspoon freshly ground black pepper
- 3/4 cup alfalfa sprouts
- 1 tablespoon chopped fresh flat-leaf parsley
- 1 tablespoon hulled pumpkin seeds
- 1 tablespoon hulled sunflower seeds

Directions:
1. In a medium bowl, whisk eggs.
2. Heat oil in a medium skillet over medium heat. Swirl oil to coat skillet. Add eggs to skillet and cook for 1 minute. Stir gently until eggs are completely cooked, about 1 minute more. Move scrambled eggs to a plate and cover to keep warm.
3. Add diced tomato to skillet and sauté over medium heat 3–5 minutes. Season with salt and pepper.
4. Divide eggs evenly onto four breakfast plates. Top eggs with tomatoes and sprouts, sprinkle with parsley and seeds, and serve.

Nutrition Info:
- Calories: 185,Fat: 13g,Protein: 14g,Sodium: 290mg,Carbohydrates: 3.

Savory Muffins

Servings: 12 | Cooking Time: 25 Minutes

Ingredients:
- ¼ cup quinoa, boiled in ½ cup water
- 1 cup oat flour
- ¼ cup corn flour
- ¼ tsp cinnamon
- Pinch of salt
- Pinch of pepper
- 3 eggs
- ½ cup lactose-free or Greek yogurt
- 2 cups zucchini, grated
- ⅓ cup baby spinach, chopped
- A few sprigs of rosemary
- ¼ cup walnuts, chopped
- ½ lemon, zested

Directions:
1. Preheat the oven to 350°F and grease a 12-hole muffin pan.
2. In a saucepan, cook the quinoa in water for 15 minutes, then drain the excess water and let cool.
3. In a bowl, mix the dry ingredients together.
4. In a larger bowl, whisk the eggs and yogurt together, then add in the zucchini, spinach, nuts, spices, lemon zest, and quinoa slowly.
5. Add the bowl of dry ingredients to the larger bowl and mix well. Spoon the batter into muffin tins and bake for 25 minutes.

Nutrition Info:
- 120g Calories, 4g Total fat, 0.8g Saturated fat, 15g Carbohydrates, 1.5 g Fiber, 4.9g Protein, 0.5g Sodium.

Rhubarb Ginger Granola Bowl

Servings: 4 | Cooking Time: 30 Minutes

Ingredients:
- Yogurt
- 1 ½ cups chopped rhubarb
- 1 tbsp grated ginger
- ½ tbsp lemon juice
- 4 tbsp maple syrup
- Pinch of salt
- 2 cups Greek yogurt
- Granola
- ½ cup pumpkin seeds
- ¾ cup chopped nuts (low-FODMAP-approved)
- 2 tbsp melted coconut oil
- 1 tsp ground ginger
- ¼ tsp cinnamon
- Pinch of salt

Directions:
1. Preheat the oven to 350°F.
2. For the yogurt, in a small pot over medium heat, add chopped rhubarb, ginger, lemon juice, and 2 tablespoons of maple syrup. Stir the mixture occasionally until it begins to simmer, ensuring the bottom of the pot does not burn. Once the mixture has thickened to a purée consistency, mix in the other 2 tablespoons of maple syrup. Place the mixture into a bowl to cool.
3. Place the granola ingredients into a separate bowl and mix until the coconut oil coats everything. Move the mix onto a non-stick baking tray and place in the oven for 10-15 minutes, stirring halfway.
4. Once all components are ready, fold the rhubarb purée into the yogurt and sprinkle the granola over top. The yogurt can be stored in the fridge and the granola in a Tupperware.
5. Add a low-FODMAP-approved topping if desired.

Nutrition Info:
- 593g Calories, 4g Total fat, 1.5g Saturated fat, 32g Carbohydrates, 4 g Fiber, 20g Protein, 19g Sodium.

Basil Vinaigrette Salad Dressing

Servings: 100 | Cooking Time: 5 Minutes

Ingredients:
- 1 cup olive oil
- ½ cup white vinegar
- 1 tbsp basil, shredded
- 1 tbsp garlic-infused oil
- Pinch of salt
- Pinch of pepper

Directions:
1. In a bottle with a lid, add all the ingredients.
2. Shake the bottle to mix and then refrigerate.

Nutrition Info:
- 20g Calories, 2.4g Total fat, 0.3g Saturated fat, 0g Carbohydrates, 0 g Fiber, 0g Protein, 0g Sodium.

Ginger-berry Rice Milk Smoothie

Servings: 2 | Cooking Time: None

Ingredients:
- 2 cups frozen strawberries, blueberries, or raspberries
- 1 cup unsweetened rice milk
- 2 tablespoons maple syrup
- 2 teaspoons finely grated fresh ginger
- 2 teaspoons lemon juice

Directions:
1. Place all of the ingredients in a blender and blend until smooth.
2. Serve immediately.

Nutrition Info:
- Calories: 162; Protein: 2g; Total Fat: 2g; Saturated Fat: 0g; Carbohydrates: 37g; Fiber: 8g;

Easy Breakfast Sausage

Servings: 4 | Cooking Time: 8 Minutes

Ingredients:
- 1 pound ground pork
- 1 teaspoon ground sage
- ½ teaspoon sea salt
- ⅛ teaspoon red pepper flakes
- ⅛ teaspoon freshly ground black pepper
- Nonstick cooking spray

Directions:
1. In a large bowl, mix the pork, sage, salt, red pepper flakes, and pepper. Form the mixture into 8 patties.
2. Spray a large nonstick skillet with cooking spray and place it over medium-high heat.
3. Add the sausage patties and cook for about 4 minutes per side, until browned on both sides.

Nutrition Info:
- Calories: 163; Total Fat: 4g; Saturated Fat: 1g; Carbohydrates: <1g; Fiber: 0g; Sodium: 299mg; Protein: 30g

Blueberry, Lime, And Coconut Smoothie

Servings: 2 | Cooking Time: 5 Minutes

Ingredients:
- ½ cup blueberries, fresh or frozen
- 2 tbsp coconut flakes
- 2 tbsp lime juice
- ⅔ cup FODMAP-approved yogurt or vegan yogurt
- 1 tsp chia seeds
- 2 tbsp water
- Ice, when using fresh blueberries (Approximately 6 cubes, depending on the desired texture)

Directions:
1. Blend all ingredients together until frothy.

Nutrition Info:
- 186g Calories, 13.5g Total fat, 5g Saturated fat, 14g Carbohydrates, 3 g Fiber, 4.5g Protein, 8.5g Sodium.

Chia Seed Carrot Cake Pudding

Servings: 2 | Cooking Time: None

Ingredients:
- ¾ cup unsweetened rice milk
- ½ cup chopped carrots
- 3 tablespoons chia seeds, divided
- 2 tablespoons maple syrup
- ½ teaspoon vanilla
- ½ teaspoon cinnamon
- ¼ teaspoon ground ginger
- ⅛ teaspoon ground cloves
- Pinch nutmeg

Directions:
1. Place the rice milk, carrots, 2 tablespoons of the chia seeds, maple syrup, vanilla, cinnamon, ginger, cloves, and nutmeg in a blender and blend until smooth. Add the remaining tablespoon of chia seeds and pulse just to incorporate.
2. Pour the mixture into two custard cups or bowls, cover, and refrigerate overnight. Serve chilled.

Nutrition Info:
- Calories: 135; Protein: 3g; Total Fat: 5g; Saturated Fat: 0g; Carbohydrates: 26g; Fiber: 8g; Sodium: 88mg;

Pb&j Smoothie

Servings: 2 | Cooking Time: 0 Minutes

Ingredients:
- 3 cups unsweetened almond milk
- 1 cup sliced strawberries, fresh or frozen
- 1 cup crushed ice
- ¼ cup sugar-free natural peanut butter
- 3 tablespoons chia seeds or ground flaxseed
- 1 packet stevia (optional)

Directions:
1. In a blender, combine the almond milk, strawberries, ice, peanut butter, chia seeds or flaxseed, and stevia (if using).
2. Blend until smooth.

Nutrition Info:
- Calories: 328; Total Fat: 25g; Saturated Fat: 4g; Carbohydrates: 18g; Fiber: 8g; Sodium: 422mg; Protein: 12g

Strawberry Smoothie

Servings: 1 | Cooking Time: 3 Minutes

Ingredients:
- ½ cup FODMAP-approved milk (almond milk is recommended)
- ⅔ cup strawberries, fresh or frozen
- ¼ cup lactose-free yogurt or vegan yogurt
- 1 ½ tsp protein powder
- 1 tsp chia seeds
- ½ tbsp maple syrup
- 1 tsp lemon juice
- ¼ tsp vanilla extract
- 6 ice cubes (only when using fresh strawberries)

Directions:
1. Cut the strawberries into halves or quarters. If using frozen strawberries, it is recommended to cut them the day before.
2. Put ingredients into a blender and blend until smooth. If the mixture gets too thick, add a small amount of hot water and continue blending.
3. It is best drunk immediately.

Nutrition Info:
- 308g Calories, 10.3g Total fat, 1.4g Saturated fat, 1.4g Carbohydrates, 5.9 g Fiber, 5.4g Protein, 30.9g Sodium.

Melon And Yogurt Parfait

Servings: 2 | Cooking Time: 0 Minutes

Ingredients:
- 2 cups chopped honeydew melon, divided
- 2 cups plain, unsweetened, lactose-free yogurt
- ¼ cup macadamia nuts, chopped

Directions:
1. In each of two medium parfait glasses or bowls, place ½ cup honeydew melon.
2. Layer a ½ cup yogurt on top of the melon.
3. Top each with 2 tablespoons macadamia nuts.
4. Repeat with the remaining ingredients.

Nutrition Info:
- Calories: 356; Total Fat: 16g; Saturated Fat: 5g; Carbohydrates: 35g; Fiber: 3g; Sodium: 203mg; Protein: 16g

Crêpes With Cheese Sauce

Servings: 4 | Cooking Time: x

Ingredients:
- CRÊPES
- ¾ cup (100 g) superfine white rice flour
- ½ cup (75 g) cornstarch
- ⅓ cup (30 g) soy flour
- ¾ teaspoon baking soda
- 2 large eggs, lightly beaten
- 1½ cups (375 ml) low-fat milk, lactose-free milk, or suitable plant-based milk
- 3 tablespoons (45 g) salted butter, melted
- Nonstick cooking spray
- CHEESE SAUCE
- 2 cups (500 ml) low-fat milk, lactose-free milk, or suitable plant-based milk
- 2 heaping tablespoons cornstarch
- 2 cups (240 g) grated reduced-fat cheddar
- Salt and freshly ground black pepper
- HAM AND SPINACH FILLING (pictured)
- Olive oil, for pan-frying
- 8 ounces (225 g) baby spinach leaves (8 cups), rinsed and dried
- 8 ounces (225 g) thinly sliced gluten-free smoked ham
- TEMPEH AND RICE FILLING
- ½ tablespoon garlic-infused olive oil
- 12 ounces (360 g) crumbled gluten-free tempeh
- ½ teaspoon smoked paprika
- Leaves from 4 thyme sprigs
- ¾ cup (140 g) cooked white rice
- 2 medium ripe tomatoes, peeled, seeded, and roughly chopped
- ½ teaspoon olive oil
- Splash of balsamic vinegar
- Salt and freshly ground black pepper to taste
- ¼ cup (40 g) pine nuts

Directions:
1. To make the crêpes, sift the rice flour, cornstarch, soy flour, and baking soda three times into a large bowl (or whisk in the bowl until well combined). Make a well in the middle, add the eggs and milk, and blend to form a smooth batter. Stir in the melted butter. Cover with plastic wrap and set aside for 20 minutes.
2. Heat a heavy-bottomed frying pan or crêpe pan over medium heat and spray well with cooking spray. Pour about ¼ cup (60 ml) batter into the warmed pan and tilt to coat the bottom thinly. Cook until bubbles start to appear, then carefully turn the crêpe over and briefly cook the other side. Transfer to a platter and cover loosely with foil to keep warm while you repeat with the remaining batter (to make 8 crêpes in total) and make the cheese sauce.
3. To make the cheese sauce, blend ¼ cup (60 ml) of the milk with the cornstarch to make a paste. Add the remaining milk, whisking well to avoid any lumps. Pour the mixture into a small saucepan and stir over medium heat until thickened. (Don't let it boil.) Add the cheddar and stir until melted. Season to taste with salt and pepper. Keep warm while you prepare the filling of your choice.
4. To make the ham and spinach filling, heat the olive oil in a large frying pan over medium heat. Add the spinach and stir to coat in the oil. Cover the pan and cook for about 1 minute, then uncover, stir, cover again, and continue to cook until just wilted, about 1 minute more. Divide the spinach evenly between the crêpes and top with the sliced ham.
5. To make the tempeh and rice filling, heat the garlic-infused oil in a large frying pan over medium-high heat. Add the crumbled tempeh, smoked paprika, and thyme and sauté until browned and crisp, about 7 minutes. Add the rice and continue to sauté until the rice is warmed through. Remove from the heat and stir in the tomatoes, olive oil, balsamic vinegar, and salt and pepper. Divide the filling evenly between the crêpes and top each with a sprinkle of pine nuts.
6. Top the crêpes with a drizzle of the cheese sauce and your choice of filling and fold to enclose. Serve with the remaining cheese sauce and a final grinding of pepper.

Nutrition Info:
- : 676 calories, 36 g protein, 31 g total fat, 65 g carbohydrates, 651 mg sodiu.

Basil Omelet With Smashed Tomato

Servings: 2 | Cooking Time: 10 Minutes

Ingredients:
- 2 tomatoes, halved
- 3 eggs
- 1 tbsp chives, chopped
- ¼ cup shredded mozzarella cheese (or other FODMAP-approved cheese)
- 1-2 basil leaves, chopped finely
- Pepper

Directions:
1. Break the eggs into a bowl and add a splash of water.

Whisk the mixture with a fork and add the chives and a pinch of pepper. Set aside.

2. Place the halved tomatoes on til in a hot skillet on the stove or onto a hot grill on low to medium heat. Turn occasionally until they are starting to char, then remove them and place them on plates. Squish slightly so that the juices are released.

3. Take the egg mixture and whisk it slightly before pouring it into a hot pan on medium heat. Leave the mixture for a few seconds before gently stirring the uncooked egg until it is cooked but still slightly loose.

4. Place the cheese and a basil leaf on one half of the egg and then gently fold the omelet in half. Let it cook for another minute. Once it is cooked, cut the omelet in half and serve with the tomato.

Nutrition Info:
- 175.5g Calories, 10.5g Total fat, 48g Saturated fat, 6g Carbohydrates, 1.5 g Fiber, 14.5g Protein, 4g Sodium.

Cinnamon Spice Granola

Servings:8 | Cooking Time:x

Ingredients:
- 2 cups quick-cooking oats
- 1 cup walnut pieces
- 1 teaspoon ground cinnamon
- 1/2 teaspoon ground nutmeg
- 1/4 teaspoon ground cloves
- 3 tablespoons light brown sugar
- 1/4 cup maple syrup
- 1/4 cup safflower oil

Directions:
1. Preheat oven to 350°F.
2. Combine all ingredients in a large bowl.
3. Spread mixture in an even layer on a baking sheet and bake 20 minutes; stir once halfway through baking.
4. Allow to cool before serving.

Nutrition Info:
- Calories: 280,Fat: 17g,Protein: 5g,Sodium: 4mg,Carbohydrates: 28.

Banana Toast

Servings:2 | Cooking Time: 5 Minutes

Ingredients:
- 4 gluten-free sandwich bread slices
- 1 ripe banana
- 1/2 teaspoon ground cinnamon

Directions:
1. Toast the bread to your desired doneness.
2. In a small bowl, mash the banana with the cinnamon and spread it on the toast.

Nutrition Info:
- Calories:102; Total Fat: <1g; Saturated Fat: 0g; Carbohydrates: 23g; Fiber: 2g; Sodium: 123mg; Protein: 2g

Breakfast Tortillas

Servings:4 | Cooking Time: 10 Minutes

Ingredients:
- 4 corn tortillas
- 4 eggs
- 1/4 cup macadamia nuts
- 1 cup mozzarella cheese, grated
- 1 cup Greek yogurt
- 4 tomatoes, diced

Directions:
1. Boil the uncracked eggs in simmering water for 5 1/2 minutes, then place in cold water to stop cooking. Peel when they have cooled.
2. Heat tortillas on both sides for 20 seconds in a pan over medium heat. Place in an airtight container and cover with a dry cloth while heating the rest of the tortillas.
3. Spread the yogurt over the tortillas and add the cheese and tomatoes. Cut the eggs in half before adding them to the tortilla. Season to taste.

Nutrition Info:
- 373g Calories, 19.5g Total fat, 9.75g Saturated fat, 19.75g Carbohydrates, 3.75 g Fiber, 19.5g Protein, 6g Sodium.

Banana Oatcakes

Servings:4 | Cooking Time: 32 Minutes

Ingredients:
- 1 unripe banana
- 1 egg
- 1/2 cup rice milk
- 1 tbsp Greek yogurt
- 1 1/2 cups rolled oats
- 1/3 cup oat flour
- 2 tsp cinnamon
- Pinch of salt

Directions:
1. Mash the banana in a bowl and add the egg, milk, and yogurt, whisking after each ingredient. Next, add the dry ingredients, making sure to mix thoroughly.
2. Let the mixture rest for 15-30 minutes.
3. Grease a pan with low-FODMAP-approved oil and place it on medium heat.
4. Pour 1/4 of the batter into the pan and flip when it begins bubbling. Remove the oatcake when it is golden brown on both sides.
5. Repeat 3 more times until you have 4 oatcakes.
6. Add a low-FODMAP-approved topping if desired.

Nutrition Info:
- 530g Calories, 12.5g Total fat, 2.75g Saturated fat, 80g Carbohydrates, 14.5 g Fiber, 21.25g Protein, 5.5g Sodium.

Egg Wraps

Servings:4 | Cooking Time: 5 Minutes

Ingredients:
- Oil to grease the pan (from the approved food list: avocado, olive, or sunflower)
- 4-8 eggs
- Pinch of salt
- Pepper

Directions:
1. Grease a non-stick pan with oil then place over medium heat to warm.
2. Whisk the egg in a bowl and pour it into the pan, ensuring it is spread evenly. Add in salt and pepper to taste.
3. Cook for 30-60 seconds on each side; gently flip when the edges on the first side are cooked.
4. Place on a plate to cool and repeat with the remainder of the eggs.

Nutrition Info:
- 414g Calories, 33g Total fat, 8g Saturated fat, 2g Carbohydrates, 0 g Fiber, 25g Protein, 2g Sodium.

Amaranth Breakfast

Servings:4 | Cooking Time:x

Ingredients:
- 1 cup amaranth seeds
- 3 cups water
- 2 teaspoons ground cinnamon
- 1 tablespoon pure vanilla extract
- 1/4 cup shelled pecans, lightly chopped

Directions:
1. Heat a heavy-bottomed saucepan over medium heat and add amaranth. Toast amaranth, stirring occasionally for 5 minutes until fragrant.
2. Pour in 3 cups water and bring to a boil. Lower heat and add cinnamon and vanilla. Cover, then simmer for 20 minutes, stirring occasionally.
3. While amaranth is simmering, place pecans under broiler for 4 minutes to toast.
4. When amaranth has finished cooking, give it a good stir and remove from heat. Serve in bowls topped with the pecans.

Nutrition Info:
- Calories: 230,Fat: 5g,Protein: 6g,Sodium: 5mg,Carbohydrates: 41.

Crispy Noodle Cakes With Chili Sauce

Servings:16 | Cooking Time:x

Ingredients:
- 1 pound (450 g) dried flat rice noodles (¼ inch/5 mm wide), broken into 2- to 4-inch (5 to 10 cm) lengths
- 3 to 4 heaping tablespoons chopped cilantro
- 2 teaspoons grated ginger
- ½ teaspoon Chinese five-spice powder
- 3 large eggs, lightly beaten
- 2 tablespoons sesame oil
- 2 teaspoons garlic-infused olive oil
- ⅓ cup (80 ml) gluten-free sweet red chili sauce*
- 2 heaping tablespoons cornstarch
- Salt
- Nonstick cooking spray
- CHILI SAUCE
- ½ cup (125 ml) gluten-free sweet red chili sauce*
- 1 heaping tablespoon tomato puree
- ½ teaspoon gluten-free soy sauce

Directions:
1. Fill a large bowl with hot water. Add the noodles and soak for 4 to 5 minutes, until softened. Drain, then rinse under cold water and place back in the bowl. Add the cilantro, ginger, five-spice powder, eggs, sesame oil, garlic-infused oil, chili sauce, cornstarch, and salt and mix until well combined.
2. Heat a large heavy-bottomed frying pan over medium heat. Spray the pan and inside of the egg rings with the cooking spray (use as many rings as will fit comfortably in the pan).
3. Spoon enough noodle mixture into each ring to fill it without overflowing. Cook for 2 to 3 minutes on each side, until golden brown. Remove from the pan and run a knife around the inside of each ring to remove the noodle cakes. Set aside on a plate and cover loosely with foil to keep warm while you make the remaining cakes.
4. For the chili sauce, combine all the ingredients in a bowl.
5. Serve the warm noodle cakes with the chili sauce.

Nutrition Info:
- : 59 calories,1 g protein,3 g total fat,6 g carbohydrates,459 mg sodiu.

Low-FODMAP Diet Cookbook

Coconut Cacao Hazelnut Smoothie Bowl

Servings:1 | Cooking Time:x

Ingredients:
- 1 tablespoon shredded unsweetened coconut
- 1 cup unsweetened almond milk
- 1 frozen medium banana
- 2 teaspoons raw unsweetened cacao powder
- 1/2 tablespoon maple syrup
- 1/8 teaspoon sea salt
- 1/2 cup ice
- 5 hazelnuts, chopped
- 1 tablespoon pumpkin seeds

Directions:

1. Toast coconut in a small skillet over medium heat, stirring frequently until flakes are golden brown. Set aside.
2. Add milk, banana, cacao, maple syrup, and salt to blender with ice and blend until smooth. Add more ice if necessary to make mixture thick and icy.
3. Pour mixture into a serving bowl and top with hazelnuts, pumpkin seeds, and toasted coconut.

Nutrition Info:
- Calories: 380,Fat: 15g,Protein: 13g,Sodium: 423mg,Carbohydrates: 54.

Bacon And Zucchini Crustless Quiche

Servings:8 | Cooking Time:x

Ingredients:
- 10 bacon slices, at room temperature
- 2 large zucchini, grated
- 1½ cups (6 ounces/180 g) grated cheddar
- 2 tablespoons canola oil
- 6 large eggs, lightly beaten
- Salt and freshly ground black pepper
- Green salad, for serving (optional)

Directions:

1. Preheat the oven to 350°F (170°C). Grease a 9-inch quiche dish or pie pan and line with a parchment paper circle. Line a plate with paper towels.
2. Add the bacon to an unheated skillet and turn the heat to medium. Cook, turning occasionally, for about 10 minutes, or until crispy. Transfer to the prepared plate to drain. When the bacon is cool enough to handle, break into small pieces.
3. Combine the bacon, zucchini, cheese, oil, and eggs in a large bowl. Season with salt and pepper. Pour into the baking dish and bake for 20 to 25 minutes, until firm and golden brown. Remove from the oven and let stand for 5 minutes before slicing. Serve it warm or cold—it's delicious either way—with a green salad, if desired.

Nutrition Info:
- : 258 calories,16 g protein,20 g total fat,3 g carbohydrates,665 mg sodiu.

High-fiber Muffins With Zucchini And Sunflower Seeds

Servings:1 | Cooking Time:x

Ingredients:
- ½ cup (75 g) cornstarch
- ½ cup (45 g) soy flour
- 2 teaspoons gluten-free baking powder
- 1 teaspoon baking soda
- 1 teaspoon xanthan gum or guar gum
- 5 tablespoons (75 g) salted butter, melted
- ½ cup (125 ml) low-fat milk, lactose-free milk, or suitable plant-based milk
- ¾ cup (200 g) gluten-free low-fat plain yogurt
- 3 large eggs
- ¾ cup (60 g) finely grated Parmesan
- ½ medium zucchini, grated
- ½ cup (75 g) roasted unsalted sunflower seeds
- ½ cup (60 g) rice bran
- ¼ cup (25 g) walnuts, crushed
- ¼ teaspoon freshly grated nutmeg
- Pinch of salt and freshly ground black pepper

Directions:

1. Preheat the oven to 325°F (170°C) and line a 12-cup muffin pan with paper liners.
2. Sift the rice flour, cornstarch, soy flour, baking powder, baking soda, and xanthan gum three times into a large bowl (or whisk in the bowl until well combined).
3. Combine the melted butter, milk, yogurt, eggs, Parmesan, zucchini, sunflower seeds, rice bran, walnuts, nutmeg, and salt and pepper in a medium bowl and mix well. Add the flour mixture and mix with a wooden spoon for 2 to 3 minutes (be careful not to overmix). Pour the batter evenly into the muffin cups until they are two-thirds full.
4. Bake for 15 to 20 minutes, until firm to the touch and a toothpick inserted into the center of a muffin comes out clean. Cool in the pan for 5 minutes, then turn out onto a wire rack to cool completely.

Nutrition Info:
- : 243 calories,9 g protein,14 g total fat,22 g carbohydrates,368 mg sodiu.

Blueberry Lime Smoothie

Servings:1 | Cooking Time: 3 Minutes

Ingredients:
- ½ cup blueberries, fresh or frozen
- 2 tbsp coconut flakes
- 2 tbsp lime juice, fresh
- ½ cup Greek or lactose-free yogurt
- 1 tsp chia seeds
- 2 tbsp water
- Ice (only if using fresh blueberries and if you want a thicker consistency)

Directions:

1. Place ingredients in a blender and mix until it starts to look frothy.

Nutrition Info:
- 319g Calories, 23g Total fat, 7g Saturated fat, 26g Carbohydrates, 6 g Fiber, 7g Protein, 15g Sodium.

Crunchy Granola

Servings:12 | Cooking Time:x

Ingredients:
- 4 cups gluten-free rolled oats
- 1/2 cup sliced almonds
- 1 cup hulled sunflower seeds
- 1/2 cup pure maple syrup
- 3 tablespoons unrefined coconut oil, liquefied
- 2 teaspoons pure vanilla extract
- 2 teaspoons ground cinnamon
- 1/2 teaspoon sea salt

Directions:
1. Preheat oven to 325°F.
2. Mix all ingredients in a large bowl. Transfer mixture to a baking sheet lined with parchment paper.
3. Cook for 50 minutes, stirring every 10–15 minutes.

Nutrition Info:
- Calories: 260,Fat: 13g,Protein: 7g,Sodium: 100mg,Carbohydrates: 31.

Carrot Cake Porridge

Servings:4 | Cooking Time: 20 Minutes

Ingredients:
- 1 cup oats
- 3 cups water
- 2 medium carrots, grated
- 1 tsp cinnamon
- 1 ½ tbsp flax seeds
- ¼ cup cranberries, dried
- ¼ cup walnuts
- ½ cup almond milk
- 1 tsp maple syrup

Directions:
1. Add the oats and water to a pot over medium heat. As it comes to a boil, turn the heat down and stir the carrots and cinnamon into the pot.
2. Cook for 10-12 minutes, until you reach the desired texture. Add the cranberries and nuts before serving.

Nutrition Info:
- 290g Calories, 9.6g Total fat, 2g Saturated fat, 29.5g Carbohydrates, 5.6 g Fiber, 9.6g Protein, 12.3g Sodium.

Chicken Liver Pâté With Pepper And Sage

Servings:12 | Cooking Time:x

Ingredients:
- 8 tablespoons (1 stick/113 g) salted butter, plus 3 tablespoons (45 g), melted
- 1 tablespoon garlic-infused olive oil
- 1 tablespoon olive oil
- 1 teaspoon finely chopped sage, plus more leaves for garnish
- 17 ounces (500 g) chicken livers, rinsed and trimmed (about 10 livers)
- 1 heaping tablespoon freshly ground black pepper
- ½ cup (125 ml) light cream
- Gluten-free crackers, for serving

Directions:
1. Combine the 8 tablespoons butter, garlic-infused oil, and olive oil in a medium saucepan over medium heat. Add the sage and cook for 2 to 3 minutes, stirring regularly. Add the chicken livers and cook until just browned. Remove from the heat and stir in the pepper and cream. Puree with an immersion blender or in a food processor until smooth. Add the melted butter and blend until combined.
2. Pour into six 4-ounce (125 ml) ramekins or one 3-cup (700 ml) mold and garnish with the sage leaves. Cover and refrigerate for 3 hours or until set.
3. Serve with crackers.

Nutrition Info:
- : 185 calories,8 g protein,16 g total fat,2 g carbohydrates,144 mg sodiu.

Breakfast Ratatouille With Poached Eggs

Servings:4 | Cooking Time: 40 Minutes

Ingredients:
- 2 tablespoons butter
- 1 medium eggplant, diced
- 4 medium tomatoes, peeled, seeded, and diced
- 1 red bell pepper, diced
- 1 green bell pepper, diced
- 2 medium zucchini, diced
- ½ cup halved artichoke hearts
- 1 jalapeño, diced
- 2 tablespoons chopped fresh thyme
- 1 tablespoon chopped fresh oregano
- ¼ cup chopped parsley
- ½ cup homemade (onion- and garlic-free) chicken or vegetable broth
- 1 teaspoon salt
- ½ teaspoon freshly ground pepper
- 4 eggs
- 2 ounces freshly grated Parmesan cheese

Directions:
1. Heat the butter in a large skillet over medium-high heat.

Add the eggplant and cook, stirring occasionally, for about 10 minutes, until the eggplant is tender. Add the tomatoes and cook for about 5 minutes, until the tomatoes have begun to break down.
2. Add the bell peppers, zucchini, artichoke hearts, jalapeño, thyme, oregano, and parsley. Stir to mix. Add the broth, salt, and pepper, and bring to a boil. Cover, reduce the heat to low, and simmer for about 20 minutes, until the liquid has evaporated and the vegetables are tender.
3. While the vegetables are cooking, poach the eggs. Bring a pan of water about 3 inches deep to a boil over high heat. Reduce the heat to low, carefully break the eggs into the water, and simmer for 4 minutes.
4. To serve, ladle the vegetable mixture into 4 serving bowls, top each with a poached egg, and sprinkle the cheese over the top. Serve hot.

Nutrition Info:
- Calories: 292; Protein: 21g; Total Fat: 15g; Saturated Fat: 7g; Carbohydrates: 24g; Fiber: 10g; Sodium: 819mg;

Quinoa Porridge

Servings:2 | Cooking Time: 25 Minutes

Ingredients:
- ½ cup quinoa
- 1 tsp oil (FODMAP-approved)
- 1 cup water
- ¾ cup milk even vegetable milk(FODMAP-approved)
- ¼ tsp cinnamon
- 2 tbsp maple syrup
- 1 cup berries (FODMAP-approved)

Directions:
1. Rinse the quinoa under cold water for two minutes using a fine sieve and then transfer it to a medium saucepan with oil. Toast the quinoa until the water has evaporated.
2. Add water to the saucepan and bring to a boil. Once the water starts boiling, turn the heat down to the lowest setting and cover with a lid. Cook for 12-15 minutes until the quinoa is fluffy. Drain the excess water and place the quinoa back into the saucepan.
3. Mix the cinnamon, milk, and syrup into the quinoa. If the milk evaporates, add a small amount as needed. Let the mix simmer for 5 minutes or until the mixture is warmed through.
4. Serve the mixture in a bowl with berries on top.

Nutrition Info:
- 292g Calories, 8g Total fat, 1.5g Saturated fat, 50.5g Carbohydrates, 4.5 g Fiber, 7.5g Protein, 17g Sodium.

Chili-cheese Muffins

Servings:1 | Cooking Time:x

Ingredients:
- ½ cup (75 g) cornstarch
- ½ cup (45 g) soy flour
- 2 teaspoons gluten-free baking powder
- 1 teaspoon baking soda
- 1 teaspoon xanthan gum or guar gum
- 1 teaspoon chili powder
- 5 tablespoons (75 g) salted butter, melted
- ¾ cup (200 g) gluten-free low-fat plain yogurt
- 3 large eggs
- ¾ cup (185 ml) low-fat milk, lactose-free milk, or suitable plant-based milk
- ¾ cup (2 ounces/60 g) finely grated Parmesan
- 1 cup (4 ounces/120 g) grated cheddar
- 2 heaping tablespoons finely chopped flat-leaf parsley
- Pinch of salt and freshly ground black pepper

Directions:
1. Preheat the oven to 325°F (170°C) and line a 12-cup muffin pan with paper liners.
2. Sift the rice flour, cornstarch, soy flour, baking powder, baking soda, xanthan gum, and chili powder three times into a large bowl (or whisk in the bowl until well combined).
3. Combine the melted butter, yogurt, eggs, milk, Parmesan, cheddar, parsley, and salt and pepper in a medium bowl and mix well. Add to the flour mixture and stir with a large metal spoon until just combined. Pour the batter evenly into the muffin cups until they are two-thirds full.
4. Bake for 15 to 20 minutes, until firm to the touch and a toothpick inserted into the center of a muffin comes out clean. Cool in the pan for 5 minutes, then turn out onto a wire rack to cool completely.

Nutrition Info:
- : 184 calories,8 g protein,13 g total fat,13 g carbohydrates,374 mg sodiu.

Quinoa Breakfast Bowl With Basil "hollandaise" Sauce

Servings:4 | Cooking Time: 15 Minutes

Ingredients:
- 1 cup uncooked quinoa
- 12 ounces green beans, trimmed and cut into 1-inch pieces
- 1½ cups water
- ½ teaspoon salt
- Basil "Hollandaise" Sauce (here)

Directions:
1. In a medium saucepan, stir together the quinoa, green beans, water, and salt. Bring to a boil over medium-high heat. Reduce the heat to low, cover, and simmer for about 15 minutes, until the quinoa is tender.
2. To serve, spoon the quinoa mixture into bowls and drizzle the sauce over the top.

Nutrition Info:
- Calories: 415; Protein: 9g; Total Fat: 28g; Saturated Fat: 3g; Carbohydrates: 36g; Fiber: 6g; Sodium: 605mg;

Pesto Noodles

Servings: 2 | Cooking Time: 10 Minutes

Ingredients:
- Pesto
- ¾ cup basil, fresh
- 2 tbsp garlic-infused oil
- ¼ cup pine nuts
- 2 tbsp olive oil
- Pinch of salt
- Pinch of pepper
- ½ cup Parmesan, grated
- Noodles
- 1 cup rice noodles

Directions:
1. In a food processor, mix basil, garlic oil, and pine nuts until coarsely chopped.
2. Add the olive oil, cheese, salt, and pepper to the processor and mix until the pesto is fully mixed and smooth.
3. Cook the noodles according to the instructions on the packet. Once cooked, toss the noodles in a bowl with 3 tablespoons pesto and mix until the noodles are covered.
4. Serve!

Nutrition Info:
- 569g Calories, 50g Total fat, 5.5g Saturated fat, 26g Carbohydrates, 3 g Fiber, 6g Protein, 1.5g Sodium.

Green Dragon Smoothie Bowl

Servings: 1 | Cooking Time: x

Ingredients:
- 1/2 cup unsweetened almond milk
- 1 small (6-ounce) tub lactose-free vanilla yogurt
- 1 tablespoon suitable protein powder
- 1 teaspoon unsweetened cocoa powder
- 1/8 teaspoon Himalayan salt
- 1 cup baby spinach
- 1/2 frozen medium banana
- 1 large slice or 2 small slices dragon fruit
- 5 almonds
- 2 tablespoons shredded unsweetened coconut
- 1/2 tablespoon chia seeds

Directions:
1. Pour almond milk and yogurt into a blender and then add protein powder, cocoa powder, salt, spinach, banana, and 1 cup ice. Blend to process. Mixture should be thick and icy; add more ice if needed. Pour into a shallow bowl.
2. Top with dragon fruit, almonds, coconut, and chia seeds. Enjoy!

Nutrition Info:
- Calories: 473, Fat: 14g, Protein: 38g, Sodium: 763mg, Carbohydrates: 55.

Fried Eggs With Potato Hash

Servings: 2 | Cooking Time: 26 Minutes

Ingredients:
- 2 tablespoons Garlic Oil, plus more as needed
- 2 russet potatoes, cut into ½-inch cubes
- 3 scallions, green parts only, chopped
- ½ teaspoon sea salt, plus more for seasoning the eggs
- ¼ teaspoon freshly ground black pepper, plus more for seasoning the eggs
- 4 eggs

Directions:
1. In a large skillet over medium-high heat, heat the garlic oil until it shimmers.
2. Add the potatoes. Cook for about 20 minutes, stirring occasionally, until soft and browned.
3. Add the scallions, salt, and pepper. Cook for 1 minute more, stirring frequently. Spoon the potatoes onto two plates.
4. Return the skillet to medium heat. If the pan is dry, add a little more garlic oil and swirl it to coat the skillet (see Tip).
5. Carefully crack the eggs into the skillet and season them with a pinch of salt and pepper. Cook undisturbed for 3 to 4 minutes, until the whites solidify.
6. Turn off the heat and carefully flip the eggs so you do not break the yolk. Leave the eggs in the hot pan for 60 to 90 seconds until the surface is cooked but the yolks remain runny.
7. Serve the potatoes topped with the eggs.

Nutrition Info:
- Calories: 401; Total Fat: 23g; Saturated Fat: 5g; Carbohydrates: 36g; Fiber: 6g; Sodium: 608mg; Protein: 15g

Soups, Salads And Sides Recipes

Soups, Salads And Sides Recipes

Rice Paper "spring Rolls" With Satay Sauce

Servings: 3 (4 Rolls Per Serving) | Cooking Time:30 Minutes

Ingredients:
- Satay sauce
- 4 tbsp peanut butter
- 2 tbsp lemon juice
- 2 tbsp water
- 2 tsp brown sugar
- 1 tsp white sugar
- Rice spring rolls
- 12 rice paper wrappers
- 1 cucumber, small
- 1 carrot, large, cut into matchstick pieces
- 1 cup red cabbage, sliced finely
- ½ cup mint, fresh, chopped roughly
- ½ cup cilantro, fresh, roughly cut

Directions:
1. Prepare the satay sauce first. Soften the peanut butter in a microwaveable bowl for about 30 seconds. Place the rest of the sauce ingredients into the bowl and use a fork to mix until smooth. Add a tbsp of water if the mixture is too thick.
2. Put warm water into a large bowl. One at a time, dip a rice wrapper into the water until it softens slightly then place it on a clean, damp cloth.
3. Place a small amount of the fresh vegetables and herbs onto the bottom third of the wrapper. Do not overfill as it will affect the rolling process.
4. To roll, first, fold the small sides up like a burrito. Next, pull the bottom of the wrapper up gently over the filling. It is best to hold the end with the filling in it in your hands.
5. The rolls are best when dipped in the satay sauce.

Nutrition Info:
- 472g Cal,23.5 g Fat ,48.2 g Carbs ,24.4 g Protein.

Lemony Grilled Zucchini With Feta And Pine Nuts

Servings:4 | Cooking Time: 8 Minutes

Ingredients:
- 3 ounces feta, crumbled
- 2 tablespoons chopped fresh mint leaves
- 2 tablespoons olive oil, divided
- 1 teaspoon fresh lemon juice
- 1 teaspoon lemon zest
- 2 scallions, green parts only, thinly sliced
- 2-3 zucchini (about 1½ pounds), halved lengthwise and cut into 3-inch pieces
- 1 teaspoon salt
- 2 tablespoons toasted pine nuts

Directions:
1. In a small bowl, stir together the feta, mint, 1 tablespoon of the oil, lemon juice, lemon zest, and scallions.
2. Brush the remaining tablespoon of oil onto the zucchini and sprinkle with the salt.
3. Heat a grill or grill pan to high heat. Cook the zucchini for 3 to 4 minutes per side, until grill marks appear and the zucchini is tender. Transfer the cooked zucchini to a serving platter, and spoon the topping over the top. Sprinkle the pine nuts over the top and serve immediately.

Nutrition Info:
- Calories: 176; Protein: 3g; Total Fat: 15g; Saturated Fat: 5g; Carbohydrates: 7g; Fiber: 2g; Sodium: 836mg;

Caramelized Squash Salad With Sun-dried Tomatoes And Basil

Servings:4 | Cooking Time:x

Ingredients:
- 2 pounds 10 ounces (1.2 kg) kabocha or other suitable winter squash, peeled, seeded, and cut into ¾-inch (2 cm) cubes
- 1 eggplant, cut into ¼-inch (5 mm) slices
- ¼ cup (60 ml) olive oil
- 12 or 13 pieces (50 g) sun-dried tomatoes in oil, drained and sliced
- ½ cup (100 g) thawed frozen corn kernels
- Small handful of basil leaves, roughly chopped

Directions:
1. Preheat the oven to 350°F (180°C).
2. Spread the squash and eggplant on two separate baking sheets and brush with 2 tablespoons of the olive oil. Bake for 25 minutes or until tender and golden brown. Let cool to room temperature, then roughly chop the eggplant.
3. Combine the squash, eggplant, sun-dried tomatoes, corn, basil, and the remaining 2 tablespoons of olive oil in a large bowl. Refrigerate for 2 to 3 hours to allow the flavors to develop. Bring to room temperature before serving.

Nutrition Info:
- : 288 calories,5 g protein,15 g total fat,41 g carbohydrates,148 mg sodiu.

Roasted Squash And Chestnut Soup

Servings:4 | Cooking Time:x

Ingredients:
- 4½ pounds (2 kg) peeled, seeded, and cubed kabocha or other suitable winter squash
- 2 tablespoons olive oil
- 2 cups (500 g) unsweetened chestnut puree
- 8 cups (2 liters) gluten-free, onion-free chicken or vegeta-

ble stock*
- 2 teaspoons ground ginger
- 1 cup (250 ml) low-fat milk, lactose-free milk, or suitable plant-based milk, warmed, plus more for serving (optional)
- Salt and freshly ground black pepper

Directions:
1. Preheat the oven to 350°F (180°C).
2. Spread the squash on a baking sheet and drizzle with the olive oil. Bake, turning occasionally, for 30 to 40 minutes, until golden and cooked through.
3. Transfer the squash to a large saucepan or stockpot. Add the chestnut puree, stock, and ginger and bring to a boil. Reduce the heat and simmer over medium-low heat for 15 to 20 minutes, stirring occasionally, until the squash is tender. Let cool for about 10 minutes.
4. Add the warmed milk to the soup and puree with an immersion blender (or in batches in a regular blender) until smooth. Season to taste with salt and pepper. Finish with a swirl of extra milk (if desired) and serve.

Nutrition Info:
- : 466 calories, 9 g protein, 10 g total fat, 92 g carbohydrates, 928 mg sodiu.

Chicken And Dumplings Soup

Servings:6 | Cooking Time:x

Ingredients:
- 1 whole (3-pound) chicken
- 2 bay leaves
- 6–8 cups water
- 2 tablespoons garlic-infused olive oil
- 5 large carrots, peeled and sliced
- 2 medium stalks celery, sliced
- 1 teaspoon dried thyme
- 1/4 teaspoon salt
- 3 whole peppercorns
- 2 cups gluten-free all-purpose flour
- 1/4 teaspoon xanthan gum
- 2 teaspoons gluten-free baking powder
- 1 teaspoon plus 1 tablespoon finely chopped fresh flat-leaf parsley, divided
- 3/4 teaspoon salt
- 2 large eggs, beaten
- 2 tablespoons butter, melted
- 3/4 cup plus 2 tablespoons lactose-free milk

Directions:
1. Put whole chicken in a large pot and add bay leaves and 6–8 cups water, or enough to cover chicken. Bring to a boil and then simmer with lid on about 1 hour, skimming off any foam. After 1 hour, remove chicken and allow to cool. Keep remaining broth in pot. Once chicken is cool, peel off skin and tear meat off bones. Set meat aside.
2. Heat oil in a large saucepan and sauté carrots and celery 5 minutes.
3. Drain broth from chicken pot through a colander into another large pot or a bowl. Discard any remaining bones and bay leaves and add drained broth to pan with vegetables and add in thyme, salt, and peppercorns. Bring to a simmer.
4. To make dumplings: combine flour, xanthan gum, baking powder, 1 teaspoon parsley, and salt in a medium bowl. Add beaten eggs, butter, and milk; gently mix to combine with a spoon. Mix just until mixture comes together nicely and stays moist. (Overmixing may make dumplings too dense.)
5. Using a soupspoon, spoon out even-sized portions of dough and drop into soup. Cover soup and simmer 20 minutes.
6. Garnish with 1 tablespoon parsley and serve.

Nutrition Info:
- Calories: 530, Fat: 14g, Protein: 56g, Sodium: 856mg, Carbohydrates: 41.

Roasted Sweet Potato Salad With Spiced Lamb And Spinach

Servings:4 | Cooking Time:x

Ingredients:
- 4 small sweet potatoes, peeled (if desired) and cut into ¾-inch (2 cm) cubes (about 4½ cups/600 g)
- 1 red bell pepper, seeded and cut into quarters
- Olive oil
- 1 heaping tablespoon ground cumin
- 2 teaspoons ground coriander
- ½ teaspoon ground cardamom
- 2 teaspoons ground turmeric
- ½ teaspoon ground sumac, or ½ teaspoon paprika plus ½ teaspoon lemon zest
- 1 pound (450 g) lean lamb steak, cut into thin strips
- 8 ounces (225 g) baby spinach leaves (8 cups), rinsed and dried

Directions:
1. Preheat the oven to 350°F (180°C).
2. Place the sweet potato and bell pepper on a large baking sheet and brush with olive oil. Roast for 30 minutes or until tender and browned. Set aside to cool. When cool enough to handle, remove the skin from the bell pepper.
3. Heat a little olive oil in a medium frying pan over medium-low heat. Add the cumin, coriander, cardamom, turmeric, and sumac and heat for 1 minute or until fragrant. Add the lamb and stir to coat with the spice mix. Cook for 3 to 5 minutes, until just browned. Remove from the heat.
4. Combine the spinach, sweet potato, and bell pepper in a large bowl. Top with the lamb and any pan juices and finish with a drizzle of olive oil.

Nutrition Info:
- : 392 calories, 27 g protein, 14 g total fat, 40 g carbohydrates, 171 mg sodiu.

Orange-maple Glazed Carrots

Servings:4 | Cooking Time:20 Minutes

Ingredients:
- 2 tablespoons pure maple syrup
- 1 tablespoon extra-virgin olive oil
- Juice of 1 orange
- Zest of 1 orange
- ½ teaspoon sea salt
- ¼ teaspoon freshly ground black pepper
- 2 cups baby carrots

Directions:
1. Preheat the oven to 400°F.
2. Line a baking sheet with parchment paper and set it aside.
3. In a medium bowl, whisk together the maple syrup, olive oil, orange juice, orange zest, salt, and pepper.
4. Add the carrots and toss to coat.
5. Spread the carrots in a single layer on the prepared sheet. Roast for 20 minutes, or until browned.

Nutrition Info:
- Calories: 101,Total Fat: 4g,Carbohydrates: 17g,Sodium: 298mg,Protein: 1.

Easy Onion- And Garlic-free Chicken Stock

Servings:2 | Cooking Time:x

Ingredients:
- 1 (2-pound) ready-made rotisserie chicken
- 2 quarts cold water
- 2 medium carrots, peeled and cut into chunks
- 1 medium stalk celery with leaves, cut into chunks
- 1 large bok choy stalk with leaves, cut into chunks
- 1/2 teaspoon dried or fresh rosemary
- 1/2 teaspoon dried or fresh thyme
- 4–5 sprigs fresh parsley
- 2 dried bay leaves
- 8 whole peppercorns

Directions:
1. Remove meat from rotisserie chicken and set aside to use for sandwiches, stir-fry, chicken salad, or other recipes.
2. Place chicken carcass in a 4- to 6-quart slow cooker and make sure it is fully covered with water.
3. Place vegetables and spices in slow cooker.
4. Set slow cooker to low and cook 6–8 hours.
5. Use tongs to transfer and discard chicken bones from slow cooker. Place a large sieve over a large bowl. Drain contents from slow cooker through sieve. Discard large vegetable pieces. Skim fat from surface of stock using a large spoon.
6. Cool completely, divide into a few small glass jars or plastic containers, and refrigerate up to 1 week or freeze up to 3 months.

Nutrition Info:
- Calories: 566,Fat: 14g,Protein: 96g,Sodium: 437mg,Carbohydrates: 7.

Coconut Rice

Servings:4 | Cooking Time: 30 Minutes

Ingredients:
- 2 cups jasmine rice
- 1 cup water
- 1 (14-ounce) can light coconut milk
- 1 teaspoon salt

Directions:
1. In a medium saucepan, combine the rice, water, coconut milk, and salt, and bring to a boil over high heat. Reduce the heat to low, cover, and cook for 30 to 40 minutes, until the rice is tender and the liquid has evaporated.
2. Remove the pot from the heat and let the rice rest, without taking the lid off, for about 10 minutes. Just before serving, fluff with a fork. Serve hot.

Nutrition Info:
- Calories: 416; Protein: 7g; Total Fat: 8g; Saturated Fat: 0g; Carbohydrates: 76g; Fiber: 1g; Sodium: 610mg;

Roasted Potato Wedges

Servings:4 | Cooking Time:30 Minutes

Ingredients:
- 1 pound Yukon Gold potatoes, quartered lengthwise
- 2 tablespoons Garlic Oil
- 1 tablespoon chopped fresh rosemary leaves
- ½ teaspoon sea salt
- ¼ teaspoon freshly ground black pepper

Directions:
1. Preheat the oven to 425°F.
2. In a large bowl, toss the potatoes with the garlic oil, rosemary, salt, and pepper. Divide them between two baking sheets and spread into a single layer.
3. Bake for about 30 minutes until the potatoes are browned. Stir them once or twice and rotate the pans (switching racks) halfway through cooking.

Nutrition Info:
- Calories: 143,Total Fat: 7g,Carbohydrates: 19g,Sodium: 241mg,Protein: 2.

Mussels In Chili, Bacon, And Tomato Broth

Servings:4 | Cooking Time:x

Ingredients:
- 4 ounces (113 g) lean bacon slices, cut crosswise into thin strips
- 2 tablespoons olive oil
- 3 cups (750 ml) tomato puree
- ½ teaspoon cayenne pepper (or to taste)
- 6½ cups (1.5 liters) reduced sodium gluten-free, onion-free chicken stock*
- 5½ pounds (2.5 kg) mussels, scrubbed and debearded

- Salt and freshly ground black pepper
- Gluten-free bread, for serving

Directions:
1. In a large heavy-bottomed saucepan over medium heat, cook the bacon until just golden. Spoon out and discard any excess fat, then add the olive oil, tomato puree, cayenne, and 2 cups (500 ml) of the stock. Bring to a boil, reduce the heat to low, and simmer for 30 to 40 minutes to develop the smoky bacon flavor.
2. Add the remaining stock. Increase the heat to medium-high and bring to a boil. Add the mussels and cook, covered, for 5 to 8 minutes, until all the mussels have opened. Shake the pan to redistribute the mussels and cook for an extra minute. Shake again. Discard any unopened mussels. Season to taste with salt and pepper and serve immediately with plenty of gluten-free bread to mop up the delicious broth.

Nutrition Info:
- : 612 calories,59 g protein,26 g total fat,33 g carbohydrates,2082 mg sodiu.

Quinoa With Cherry Tomatoes, Olives, And Radishes

Servings:4 | Cooking Time: 20 Minutes

Ingredients:
- 1 cup uncooked quinoa
- 1 teaspoon salt
- ¼ cup white wine vinegar or white balsamic vinegar
- ¼ cup olive oil
- 1 cup cherry tomatoes, halved or quartered
- 1 cup pitted cured black olives, halved, quartered, or left whole if small
- 4 to 6 radishes, thinly sliced

Directions:
1. In a medium saucepan, combine the quinoa and salt with 2 cups water and bring to a boil. Reduce the heat to low, cover, and let simmer for 15 to 20 minutes, until tender.
2. Meanwhile, in a small bowl, whisk together the vinegar and olive oil. When the quinoa is cooked, immediately toss it together with the dressing in a large bowl. Add the tomatoes, olives, and radishes and toss together. Serve immediately or refrigerate, covered, for up to 3 days.

Nutrition Info:
- Calories: 309; Protein: 7g; Total Fat: 19g; Saturated Fat: 3g; Carbohydrates: 31g; Fiber: 5g; Sodium: 886mg;

Sesame Rice Noodles

Servings:4 | Cooking Time: About 10 Minutes

Ingredients:
- 1 package rice noodles, such as pad Thai noodles
- FOR THE SAUCE
- ¼ cup gluten-free soy sauce
- 3 tablespoons dark sesame oil
- 2 tablespoons rice vinegar
- 2 tablespoons sugar
- 1 tablespoon Garlic Oil (here)
- ½ teaspoon chili oil or onion- and garlic-free chili paste
- 2 tablespoons chopped cilantro (optional)

Directions:
1. Cook the noodles according to the package instructions.
2. While the noodles are cooking, make the sauce. In a small bowl, whisk together the soy sauce, sesame oil, vinegar, sugar, Garlic Oil, and chili oil or paste until well combined.
3. In a large bowl, toss the warm, cooked noodles with the sauce until well coated. Serve immediately, garnished with cilantro if desired.

Nutrition Info:
- Calories: 270; Protein: 1g; Total Fat: 11g; Saturated Fat: 2g; Carbohydrates: 40g; Fiber: 1g; Sodium: 74mg;

Chive Dip

Servings: 10 | Cooking Time:30 Minutes

Ingredients:
- 2 tbsp parsley, fresh, chopped finely
- 1 cup mayonnaise
- 2 tbsp chives, dried
- 2 tbsp oil (best with onion-infused but can be substituted with other approved oils)
- Pinch of salt
- 1 tsp lemon juice

Directions:
1. Mix the mayonnaise, oil, chives, salt, and parsley together in a bowl. Add lemon juice or herbs of choice to taste.
2. Chill in the fridge for 30 minutes and serve with approved fresh vegetables or chips.

Nutrition Info:
- 82g Cal,7.8 g Fat ,2.9 g Carbs ,0.4 g Protein.

Turkey-ginger Soup

Servings:4 | Cooking Time:17 Minutes

Ingredients:
- 2 tablespoons Garlic Oil
- 1 pound ground turkey
- 6 scallions, green parts only, chopped
- 2 carrots, chopped
- 2 tablespoons peeled, minced fresh ginger
- 7 cups Low-FODMAP Poultry Broth
- ½ teaspoon sea salt
- ⅛ teaspoon freshly ground black pepper
- 2 cups cooked brown rice

Directions:
1. In a large pot over medium-high heat, heat the garlic oil until it shimmers.
2. Add the turkey. Cook for about 5 minutes, crumbling it with the back of a spoon, until browned.
3. Add the scallions, carrots, and ginger. Cook for 3 minutes, stirring.

4. Stir in the broth, salt, and pepper. Bring to a simmer. Cook for about 7 minutes, until the carrots soften.
5. Stir in the brown rice and cook for 2 minutes more to heat through.

Nutrition Info:
- Calories: 482,Total Fat: 16g,Carbohydrates: 44g,Sodium: 610mg,Protein: 44.

Classic Coleslaw

Servings:6 | Cooking Time: None

Ingredients:
- 1 cup mayonnaise
- 3 tablespoons Dijon mustard
- 1 tablespoon white-wine vinegar
- Juice of 1 lemon
- Pinch sugar
- ½ teaspoon celery seed
- Several dashes onion- and garlic-free hot-pepper sauce
- ¾ teaspoon salt
- ½ teaspoon freshly ground black pepper
- 1 head green cabbage, shredded
- 2 carrots, grated
- 1 fresh red chile, sliced

Directions:
1. In a large bowl, combine the mayonnaise, mustard, vinegar, lemon juice, sugar, celery seed, hot sauce, salt, and pepper, and stir together.
2. Add the cabbage and carrots to the dressing, and toss together until evenly coated.
3. Cover and chill the coleslaw for at least 2 hours before serving.

Nutrition Info:
- Calories: 198; Protein: 5g; Total Fat: 14g; Saturated Fat: 2g; Carbohydrates: 19g; Fiber: 4g; Sodium: 694mg;

Blue Cheese And Arugula Salad With Red Wine Dressing

Servings:4 | Cooking Time:x

Ingredients:
- 4 handfuls of arugula
- 1 cup (50 g) snow pea shoots or bean sprouts
- 7 ounces (200 g) blue cheese, cut into small chunks
- ½ English cucumber, sliced
- 1 avocado, pitted, peeled, and sliced (optional)
- ½ green bell pepper, seeded and thinly sliced
- RED WINE DRESSING
- ¼ cup (60 ml) olive oil
- 2 tablespoons plus 2 teaspoons fresh lemon juice
- 1 tablespoon red wine vinegar
- 1 teaspoon gluten-free whole grain mustard
- 1 teaspoon sugar
- 2 heaping tablespoons chopped tarragon or flat-leaf parsley

Directions:
1. Combine the arugula, snow pea shoots, blue cheese, cucumber, avocado (if using), and bell pepper in a large bowl.
2. To make the dressing, combine all the ingredients in a small screw-top jar and shake until well mixed.
3. Just before serving, pour the dressing over the salad and gently toss to combine.

Nutrition Info:
- : 403 calories,13 g protein,36 g total fat,12 g carbohydrates,728 mg sodiu.

Bacon Mashed Potatoes

Servings:4 | Cooking Time: 15 Minutes

Ingredients:
- 1 pound new or baby potatoes, cut into 1-inch cubes
- 2 slices bacon
- ⅓ cup lactose-free milk
- ½ teaspoon salt
- ¼ teaspoon freshly ground black pepper
- ¼ cup unsalted butter
- 4 scallions, green parts only, sliced

Directions:
1. Put the potatoes in a large saucepan, cover with 2 inches of water, and bring to a boil over medium-high heat. Lower the heat to medium and cook for 10 to 12 minutes, until the potatoes are tender. Drain the potatoes and place them in a large bowl.
2. While the potatoes are cooking, cook the bacon in a large skillet over medium heat for about 4 minutes per side, until browned and crisp. Drain on paper towels, and then crumble.
3. In the large bowl, mash the potatoes with a potato masher. Add the milk, salt, pepper, and butter. Continue mashing until the potatoes are smooth, the butter is melted, and everything is well mixed. Stir in the bacon and scallions. Serve immediately.

Nutrition Info:
- Calories: 203; Protein: 5g; Total Fat: 14g; Saturated Fat: 8g; Carbohydrates: 16g; Fiber: 3g; Sodium: 479mg;

Prosciutto Di Parma Salad

Servings:2 | Cooking Time:x

Ingredients:
- For the salad:
- 2 cups mix of baby spinach and arugula
- 25 blueberries
- 15 macadamia nuts, halved
- 6 slices prosciutto di Parma
- 1/8 teaspoon sea salt
- 1 cup crumbled goat cheese
- 1/4 teaspoon freshly ground black pepper
- For the dressing:
- 1 tablespoon rice wine vinegar
- 1 tablespoon extra-virgin olive oil
- 1 tablespoon maple syrup

Directions:
1. Layer baby spinach, arugula, blueberries, nuts, and prosciutto in a medium bowl. Sprinkle with salt.
2. Make dressing by whisking together rice vinegar, oil, and maple syrup in a small bowl.
3. Pour dressing over salad and cover bowl with a lid or plastic wrap. Shake until well-coated.
4. Add crumbled goat cheese and black pepper and serve.

Nutrition Info:
- Calories: 546,Fat: 41g,Protein: 33g,Sodium: 1,461mg,Carbohydrates: 11g,Calories: 87,Fat: 7g,Protein: 0g,Sodium: 1mg,Carbohydrates: 7.

Potato Leek Soup
Servings:4 | Cooking Time:13 Minutes

Ingredients:
- 6 cups Low-FODMAP Vegetable Broth
- 5 russet potatoes, peeled and chopped
- 2 leeks, green parts only, thoroughly washed (see Tip) and chopped
- ½ teaspoon sea salt
- ⅛ teaspoon freshly ground black pepper

Directions:
1. In a large pot over medium-high heat, stir together the broth, potatoes, leeks, salt, and pepper. Bring the soup to a boil. Reduce the heat to medium and simmer the soup for about 10 minutes, until the potatoes and leeks are soft.
2. In a blender or food processor, purée the soup, in batches if needed, until smooth. For safe puréeing of hot soup, see the Tip for Carrot and Ginger Soup.

Nutrition Info:
- Calories: 234,Total Fat: <1g,Carbohydrates: 55g,Sodium: 304mg,Protein: 5.

Abundantly Happy Kale Salad
Servings:5 | Cooking Time:x

Ingredients:
- 9 large leaves curly kale, thinly shredded (ribs and stems removed)
- 1/2 teaspoon sea salt
- 3 tablespoons extra-virgin olive oil, divided
- Juice of 1 large lemon
- 1 cup shredded butter lettuce
- 1 medium stalk celery, diced
- 1 medium yellow bell pepper, seeded and diced
- 1 medium carrot, peeled and grated
- 1 tablespoon hemp seeds
- 1 tablespoon pumpkin seeds
- 1 tablespoon chopped walnuts
- 2 cups shredded common (green) cabbage
- 2 radishes, sliced very thin
- 1 cup sliced fennel bulb
- 1 cup fresh blueberries

Directions:
1. Add kale to a medium bowl and sprinkle salt and 2 tablespoons oil on top. Massage leaves with hands until leaves begin to darken and soften.
2. Add remaining oil and remaining ingredients and toss gently. Keep covered in refrigerator up to 3 days.

Nutrition Info:
- Calories: 163,Fat: 11g,Protein: 4g,Sodium: 289mg,Carbohydrates: 17.

Beetroot Dip
Servings: 6 | Cooking Time:-

Ingredients:
- 1 ¼ cups baby beetroot, canned, drained
- 1 tbsp lemon juice
- 1 cup mint leaves, unchopped
- 1 tsp cumin seeds, whole
- ½ tsp fennel seeds
- ½ tsp coriander, ground
- ½ cup coconut yogurt, or other approved yogurts

Directions:
1. In a blender or food processor, place the beetroot, lemon juice, coriander, cumin, and fennel. Add the yogurt to the mixture and mix until the dip is smooth and at the desired consistency. The dip will thicken when it is cooled in the fridge.
2. Serve with plain chips, fresh vegetables, or rice crackers.

Nutrition Info:
- 63g Cal,4.6 g Fat ,5 g Carbs ,1.1 g Protein.

Veggie Dip
Servings: 16 | Cooking Time:5 Minutes

Ingredients:
- 1 cup mayonnaise
- 2 cups Greek yogurt
- 2 cups kale, chopped finely
- 1 ½ cups bell peppers, variety of colors, chopped finely
- 2 cups water chestnuts, chopped finely
- 3 spring onions, green parts only, chopped finely
- 1 tsp garlic-infused oil
- Pinch of salt
- Fresh sliced vegetables and corn chips for serving

Directions:
1. In a bowl, mix all the ingredients well, except for the fresh sliced vegetables. Place in the fridge until serving.
2. Serve with the fresh vegetables.

Nutrition Info:
- 123g Cal,10 g Fat ,3 g Carbs ,3 g Protein.

Quinoa With Swiss Chard

Servings:4 | Cooking Time: 25 Minutes

Ingredients:
- 1 tablespoon Garlic Oil (here)
- 1 bunch Swiss chard, stems removed and leaves julienned
- 1 teaspoon ground cumin
- 1 teaspoon ground coriander
- 2 teaspoons paprika
- ½ teaspoon salt
- 1 cup quinoa
- 2 cups homemade (onion- and garlic-free) vegetable broth

Directions:
1. Heat the oil in a large skillet set over medium heat. Add the Swiss chard, cumin, coriander, paprika, salt, quinoa, and broth and bring to a boil.
2. Cover, reduce the heat to low, and cook for 20 minutes, until the liquid has evaporated and the quinoa is tender. Serve hot.

Nutrition Info:
- Calories: 207; Protein: 9g; Total Fat: 7g; Saturated Fat: 1g; Carbohydrates: 29g; Fiber: 4g; Sodium: 753mg;

Butter Lettuce Salad With Poached Egg And Bacon

Servings:4 | Cooking Time:x

Ingredients:
- 4 slices thick-cut bacon
- 1 tablespoon fresh lemon juice
- 2 teaspoons Dijon mustard
- 2 tablespoons extra-virgin olive oil
- 1/2 teaspoon freshly ground black pepper
- 1 tablespoon rice wine vinegar
- 4 large eggs
- 4 cups butter lettuce

Directions:
1. Preheat oven to 400°F.
2. Line a rimmed baking sheet with parchment paper and place bacon on top of paper. Bake 15–18 minutes or until crisp and browned, rotating baking sheet once. Drain bacon strips on a plate with paper towels. Once cool enough to handle, cut bacon into 1/2" strips.
3. In a small bowl combine lemon juice, mustard, oil, and pepper. Stir well to combine.
4. Pour cold water into a large saucepan until there is at least 4" of water. Add vinegar and bring to a boil over medium heat, then reduce heat to low.
5. Crack 1 egg into a small shallow bowl. Stir water in saucepan continuously to create a whirlpool. Gently pour egg into water. Cook 3–4 minutes until firm. Remove egg from water with a slotted spoon. Skim any remaining foam from water. Repeat with remaining eggs.
6. Place lettuce and bacon in a large salad bowl. Pour in lemon-mustard dressing. Toss well to combine. Divide among 4 plates. Gently add 1 egg to each plate and serve.

Nutrition Info:
- Calories: 223,Fat: 20g,Protein: 9g,Sodium: 324mg,Carbohydrates: 1.

Roasted Vegetable Soup

Servings:8 | Cooking Time:x

Ingredients:
- 1 recipe Roasted Vegetables (see recipe in Chapter 13)
- 1 (14.5-ounce) can diced tomatoes
- 6 cups Basic Roast Chicken Stock (see recipe in this chapter)
- 1 tablespoon chopped fresh flat-leaf parsley

Directions:
1. Place vegetables in a stockpot and add tomatoes and stock. Stir to combine. Working in batches, place vegetables in a blender or food processor. Blend until smooth. If desired, you can leave some vegetables unblended for texture.
2. Return puréed vegetables to pot. Heat on high until boiling. Lower heat and simmer, uncovered, for 20 minutes to blend flavors and heat through.
3. Serve with a garnish of chopped parsley.

Nutrition Info:
- Calories: 270,Fat: 10g,Protein: 12g,Sodium: 545mg,Carbohydrates: 34.

Zucchini Ribbon Salad With Goat Cheese, Pine Nuts, And Pomegranate

Servings:8 | Cooking Time:x

Ingredients:
- 4 large zucchini
- 1/4 teaspoon kosher salt
- 1/8 teaspoon coarse sea salt
- 1/4 cup extra-virgin olive oil
- 3 tablespoons rice wine vinegar
- Juice of 1 large lemon
- 2 tablespoons fresh parsley
- 1/4 cup pine nuts
- 1/2 cup pomegranate seeds
- 1/2 teaspoon freshly ground black pepper
- 3/4 cup crumbled goat cheese

Directions:
1. Peel zucchini and use a mandoline, a spiralizer with a straight blade, or a vegetable peeler to make thin ribbons. Place zucchini in a colander and sprinkle with kosher salt. Let sit 25–30 minutes, then lay on paper towels.
2. Meanwhile, in a large salad bowl, add oil, vinegar, lemon juice, parsley, pine nuts, pomegranate seeds, sea salt, and pepper. Add zucchini and toss well to combine. Cover with plastic wrap and refrigerate 4–6 hours.
3. Remove salad from refrigerator. Toss again. Top with goat cheese and toss gently. Serve.

Nutrition Info:

- Calories: 185, Fat: 14g, Protein: 2g, Sodium: 197mg, Carbohydrates: 16.

Roast Vegetables

Servings: 6 | Cooking Time: 45 Minutes

Ingredients:
- Vegetables
- 1 ½ cups carrot
- 1 ½ cups parsnip
- 1 ½ cups pumpkin
- 2 red bell peppers
- 1 ¾ cup potatoes
- 1 ⅓ cup baby beetroot, drained
- Pinch of salt
- Pinch of pepper
- Glaze
- 4 tbsp olive oil
- 1 ½ tbsp ginger, crushed
- 1 tbsp maple syrup

Directions:
1. Preheat the oven to 375°F and line a baking tray with parchment paper.
2. To prepare the vegetables, first, clean them and cut the carrots in half, if using large ones. Deseed the pepper and slice. Remove the skin of the pumpkin, parsnips, and potatoes before cutting into chunks. Cut the drained baby beetroots in half.
3. In the tray, place the vegetables in one layer and toss with a small amount of oil, salt, and pepper. Place in the oven.
4. The glaze is made by mixing the ingredients together in a bowl.
5. Baste the vegetables by coating them in a layer of glaze two to three times while cooking. Be sure to flip the vegetables halfway through the cooking process. Remove after 45 minutes, when they should be golden and crispy.

Nutrition Info:
- 316g Cal, 10.2 g Fat, 52.9 g Carbs, 6.1 g Protein.

Creamy Seafood Soup

Servings: 6 | Cooking Time: x

Ingredients:
- 3 tablespoons (45 g) salted butter
- 2 large carrots, diced
- ½ cup (100 g) long-grain white rice
- 5 cups (1.25 liters) gluten-free, onion-free chicken stock*
- 2 tablespoons plus 2 teaspoons fish sauce, or 4 teaspoons soy sauce plus 2 teaspoons fresh lime juice
- ½ cup (125 ml) tomato puree
- ½ fennel bulb, finely chopped
- ½ cup (125 ml) white wine (optional)
- 1 pound (450 g) raw medium shrimp, peeled and deveined
- 2 large or 5 small squid bodies, cleaned and sliced (5 ounces/150 g)
- 5 ounces (150 g) boneless, skinless firm fish fillets, cut into cubes
- 6 cooked jumbo shrimp
- 1 cup (250 ml) low-fat milk, lactose-free milk, or suitable plant-based milk
- Salt and freshly ground black pepper
- Extra virgin olive oil, to garnish (optional)

Directions:
1. Melt the butter in a large heavy-bottomed saucepan over medium heat. Add the carrots and rice and cook, stirring regularly, for 5 minutes.
2. Add the stock, fish sauce, tomato puree, fennel, and wine (if using) and stir to combine. Bring to a boil, reduce the heat to low, and simmer for 20 minutes, until the rice is tender.
3. Let cool for 10 minutes. Puree with an immersion blender (or in batches in a regular blender) until smooth.
4. Return the pan to the stove over medium heat and bring the soup to a simmer. Add the uncooked shrimp, squid, and fish and simmer for 4 to 5 minutes, until the seafood is just cooked. Add the jumbo shrimp and milk and stir until heated through and combined. Season to taste with salt and pepper, finish with a drizzle of olive oil (if desired), and serve immediately.

Nutrition Info:
- : 296 calories, 32 g protein, 9 g total fat, 17 g carbohydrates, 1300 mg sodiu.

Fennel Pomegranate Salad

Servings: 2 | Cooking Time: x

Ingredients:
- 3 small fennel bulbs, thinly sliced
- 1/4 medium stalk celery, sliced into thin slivers
- 1/2 cup coarsely chopped fresh parsley
- 1/2 cup pomegranate seeds, divided
- 1/4 cup fresh lemon juice
- 1/4 cup extra-virgin olive oil
- 1/4 teaspoon salt
- 1/2 teaspoon freshly ground black pepper
- 1/2 cup crumbled goat cheese

Directions:
1. Toss fennel, celery, parsley, and 1/4 cup pomegranate seeds in a large bowl.
2. Add lemon juice and oil and toss to coat. Add salt and pepper.
3. Serve topped with goat cheese and remaining pomegranate seeds.

Nutrition Info:
- Calories: 394, Fat: 30g, Protein: 12g, Sodium: 400mg, Carbohydrates: 23.

Kale And Red Bell Pepper Salad

Servings:4 | Cooking Time:0 Minutes

Ingredients:
- 4 cups stemmed, chopped kale, or 1 (9-ounce) bag kale salad
- 1 red bell pepper, stemmed, seeded, and chopped
- ¼ cup pepitas (hulled pumpkin seeds)
- ¼ cup Balsamic Vinaigrette

Directions:
1. In a large bowl, combine the kale, bell pepper, and pepitas.
2. Add the vinaigrette and toss to coat.

Nutrition Info:
- Calories: 149,Total Fat: 10g,Carbohydrates: 12g,Sodium: 151mg,Protein: 4.

Pesto Ham Sandwich

Servings:2 | Cooking Time:0 Minutes

Ingredients:
- 4 slices gluten-free sandwich bread, toasted
- 4 tablespoons Macadamia Spinach Pesto, divided
- 4 ounces thinly sliced prosciutto, divided
- 4 pieces jarred roasted red pepper

Directions:
1. Spread 2 bread slices with 2 tablespoons pesto each.
2. Top each with half the prosciutto and half the roasted red pepper.
3. Top with the remaining bread slices.

Nutrition Info:
- Calories: 238,Total Fat: 12g,Carbohydrates: 25g,Sodium: 790mg,Protein: 9.

Hearty Lamb Shank And Vegetable Soup

Servings:4 | Cooking Time:x

Ingredients:
- 3 tablespoons olive oil
- 1 tablespoon garlic-infused olive oil
- 2 lamb shanks (about 2 pounds/900 g)
- 1½ pounds (700 g) kabocha or other suitable winter squash, peeled, seeded, and cut into ¾-inch (2 cm) pieces
- 3 large carrots, cut into ⅓-inch (1 cm) pieces
- 3 celery stalks, cut into ⅓-inch (1 cm) slices
- 6½ cups (1.5 liters) gluten-free, onion-free beef stock*
- ⅔ cup (130 g) long-grain white rice
- Salt and freshly ground black pepper

Directions:
1. Heat the olive oil and garlic-infused oil in a large heavy-bottomed saucepan over medium heat. Add the lamb shanks and cook on all sides until lightly browned, 5 to 10 minutes total, searing for 2 to 3 minutes on each side before turning. Remove the shanks and set aside on a plate. Add the squash, carrots, and celery to the pan and cook in the remaining oil and meat juices for 2 to 3 minutes, until lightly golden.
2. Increase the heat to medium-high and return the shanks to the pan. Add the stock and rice and bring to a boil, then reduce the heat and simmer, stirring occasionally, for 50 to 60 minutes, until the meat is very tender.
3. Remove the lamb shanks, then remove the meat from the bones and shred or cut into large pieces. Discard the bones and fat. Return the lamb to the pan and stir until well combined, breaking up the squash pieces. Season well with salt and pepper and serve.

Nutrition Info:
- : 623 calories,40 g protein,30 g total fat,49 g carbohydrates,804 mg sodiu.

Kale Sesame Salad With Tamari-ginger Dressing

Servings:2 | Cooking Time:x

Ingredients:
- 1 1/2 tablespoons sesame seeds
- 4 cups shredded kale (thick ribs and stems removed)
- 3 tablespoons extra-virgin olive oil, divided
- 1 tablespoon chopped scallion, green part only
- 1/2 cup peeled and julienned carrots
- 1 tablespoon rice wine vinegar
- 1/2 tablespoon finely grated gingerroot
- 1/2 tablespoon gluten-free soy sauce (tamari)
- 1 teaspoon lime juice
- 1/16 teaspoon wheat-free asafetida powder
- 1/4 medium avocado, sliced in half
- 2 tablespoons chopped fresh basil

Directions:
1. Using a small skillet set over medium-high heat, toast sesame seeds until golden brown, about 1 minute. Stir continuously to keep seeds from burning. Set aside.
2. Place kale in a large salad bowl. Add 1 tablespoon olive oil and massage with hands until kale leaves become soft. Add scallion and carrots and toss to combine.
3. Make dressing in a small bowl by whisking together vinegar, ginger, soy sauce, lime juice, and asafetida.
4. Pour dressing over kale and stir again to combine. Divide into 2 salad bowls and top each with sesame seeds, 1 slice avocado, and 1 tablespoon basil.

Nutrition Info:
- Calories: 344,Fat: 28g,Protein: 7g,Sodium: 306mg,Carbohydrates: 21.

Philly Steak Sandwich

Servings:2 | Cooking Time:15 Minutes

Ingredients:
- 2 tablespoons Garlic Oil
- 1 green bell pepper, sliced
- 1 red bell pepper, sliced
- 6 scallions, green parts only, sliced
- 6 ounces thinly sliced deli roast beef, chopped
- 2 slices gluten-free sandwich bread, toasted
- ½ cup grated Monterey Jack cheese

Directions:
1. In a large nonstick skillet over medium-high heat, heat the garlic oil until it shimmers.
2. Add the green and red bell peppers and the scallions. Cook for about 7 minutes, stirring occasionally, until soft.
3. Add the roast beef, and cook for about 3 minutes more, until the beef is warmed through.
4. Preheat the broiler to high and adjust a rack to the top position.
5. Place the toasted bread on a baking sheet and top each with half the bell peppers and beef.
6. Sprinkle each with ¼ cup grated cheese.
7. Broil for about 3 minutes, until the cheese melts.

Nutrition Info:
- Calories: 501,Total Fat: 31g,Carbohydrates: 30g,Sodium: 641mg,Protein: 28.

Mom's Chicken Salad

Servings:4 | Cooking Time:x

Ingredients:
- 1 1/2 pounds boneless, skinless chicken breasts
- 2 cups Easy Onion- and Garlic-Free Chicken Stock (see recipe in this chapter)
- 1/8 teaspoon salt, divided
- 1/2 teaspoon dried thyme
- 1 cup Basic Mayonnaise (see Chapter 13)
- 1/2 medium stalk celery, diced
- 1 1/2 teaspoons finely chopped fresh tarragon
- 1/4 teaspoon freshly ground black pepper

Directions:
1. In a 2–4-quart saucepan with a lid, arrange chicken breasts in a single layer and set to medium-high heat. Pour in chicken stock, 1/16 teaspoon salt, and thyme. If stock is not covering chicken breasts completely, add some water.
2. Bring to a boil, then reduce heat to low and cover pot; poach chicken 8–12 minutes. Check chicken after 8 minutes. If it is opaque throughout, it is ready. An instant-read thermometer placed in thickest part of meat should register 165°F. Transfer chicken with a slotted spoon to a plate and cover with plastic wrap. Chill in refrigerator 20–30 minutes.
3. Remove chicken from plastic wrap and cut into cubes, removing any white film that might still remain.
4. Add chicken, mayonnaise, celery, tarragon, remaining salt, and pepper to a medium serving bowl. Stir well to combine. Chill in the refrigerator until ready to serve.

Nutrition Info:
- Calories: 631,Fat: 50g,Protein: 39g,Sodium: 710mg,Carbohydrates: 6.

Roman Egg Drop Soup

Servings:8 | Cooking Time:x

Ingredients:
- 8 cups Easy Onion- and Garlic-Free Chicken Stock (see recipe in this chapter)
- 1/2 teaspoon kosher salt, divided
- 4 cups packed spinach leaves, shredded
- 4 large eggs
- 1/2 cup grated Parmigiano-Reggiano, divided
- 1/2 teaspoon freshly ground black pepper
- 1/4 teaspoon ground nutmeg
- 3 tablespoons chopped fresh Italian parsley

Directions:
1. In a medium pot, bring stock to a simmer with 1/4 teaspoon salt. After 3–4 minutes, add spinach and cook until tender, about 3 minutes.
2. Meanwhile, in a medium bowl, whisk together eggs, 1/4 cup cheese, remaining 1/4 teaspoon salt, and pepper.
3. Add a 1/3 of egg mixture to stock and spinach, and continuously whisk. Add nutmeg, remaining eggs in 2 more batches, and allow soup to return to a boil. If any large clusters of eggs form, whisk until you see more shreds of eggs. Serve soup with remaining cheese and garnish with parsley.

Nutrition Info:
- Calories: 154,Fat: 7g,Protein: 12g,Sodium: 710mg,Carbohydrates: 10.

Fish And Seafood Recipes

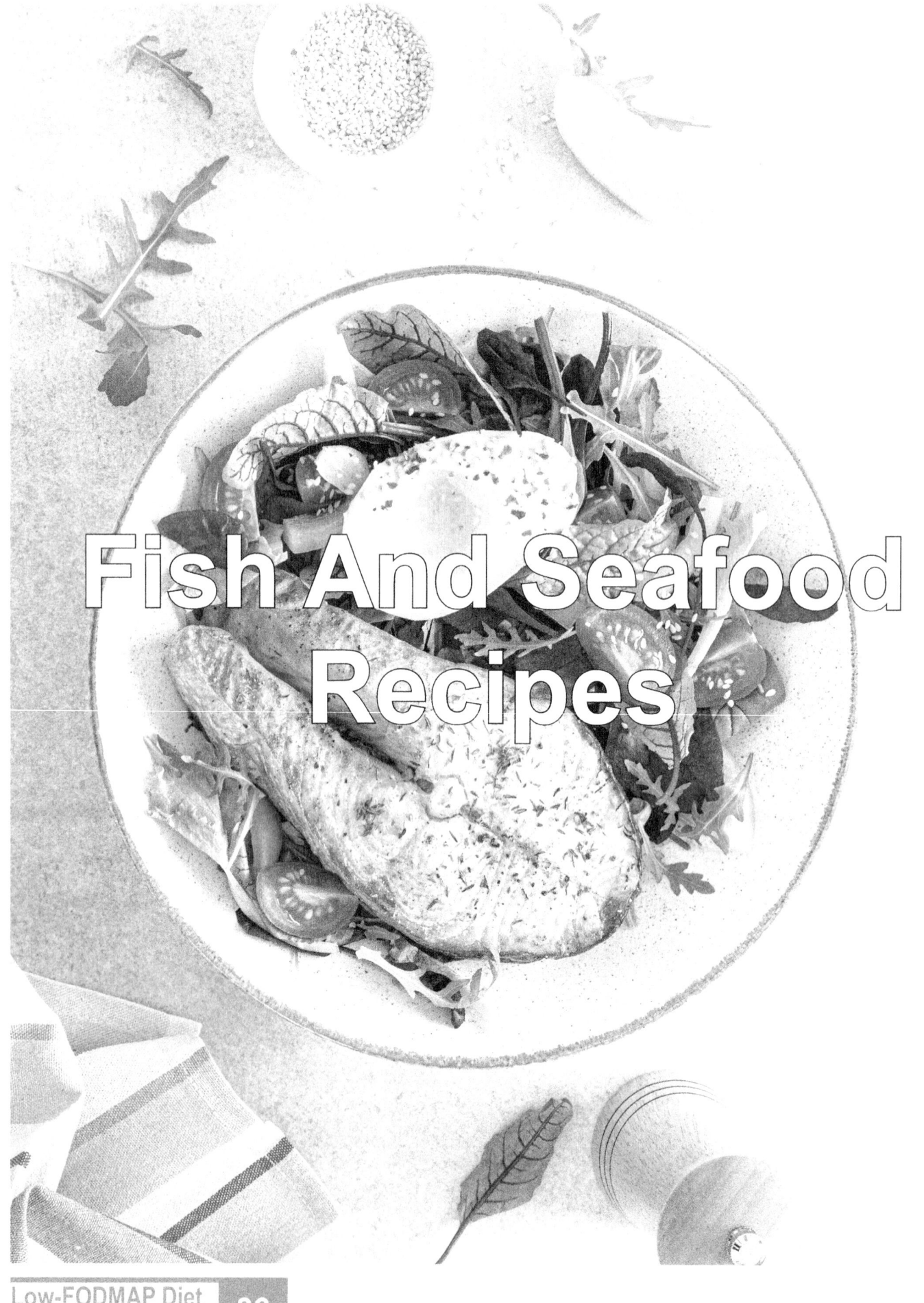

Low-FODMAP Diet Cookbook

Fish And Seafood Recipes

Summery Fish Stew
Servings:6 | Cooking Time:x

Ingredients:
- 2 slices raw bacon
- 1 cup sliced carrot
- 4 cups Seafood Stock (see recipe in Chapter 8)
- 1/2 cup dry white wine
- 1 (14.5-ounce) can fire-roasted diced tomatoes
- 1 bay leaf
- 1 teaspoon sea salt
- 1/4 teaspoon freshly ground black pepper
- 2 small red potatoes, peeled and cut into 1" pieces
- 2 pounds raw white-fleshed fish fillets, cut into 2" pieces
- 1 cup cut green beans
- 1 cup corn kernels
- 1/2 cup Whipped Cream (see recipe in Chapter 14)
- 1 tablespoon chopped fresh parsley

Directions:
1. Cook bacon in a large stockpot over medium heat. Transfer bacon to a paper towel–lined plate to cool.
2. To same pot, add carrots and sauté for 10 minutes over medium-low heat, stirring occasionally. Add stock, wine, tomatoes, bay leaf, salt, and pepper.
3. Bring just to a boil, then reduce heat and simmer for 20 minutes. Add potatoes and simmer uncovered 15 minutes. Add fish, beans, and corn; return to a simmer, stirring occasionally. Simmer uncovered 5 minutes. Remove from heat and let stand 5 minutes more, until fish is cooked through.
4. Remove and discard bay leaf. Chop and add in bacon. Stir in whipped cream.
5. Ladle stew into bowls, garnish with parsley, and serve.

Nutrition Info:
- Calories: 414,Fat: 15g,Protein: 36g,Sodium: 1,455mg,Carbohydrates: 31.

Coconut Shrimp
Servings:4 | Cooking Time:x

Ingredients:
- 1 slice gluten-free bread, toasted
- 1/2 cup unsweetened finely shredded coconut
- 1/8 teaspoon sea salt
- 1 large egg
- 1/8 teaspoon pure vanilla extract
- 16 large raw shrimp, peeled and deveined

Directions:
1. Preheat oven to 425°F. Line a baking sheet with foil and coat with coconut oil spray.
2. Add toast to food processor. Pulse until fine bread crumbs form.
3. In a flat dish, mix bread crumbs with coconut and salt.
4. In a small bowl, whisk together egg and vanilla.
5. Dip each shrimp into egg mixture, then into breadcrumb/coconut mixture. Transfer to baking sheet.
6. Bake for 5 minutes. Carefully turn each shrimp over and bake for 5 minutes more or until shrimp are fully cooked through. Serve immediately.

Nutrition Info:
- Calories: 88,Fat: 5g,Protein: 5g,Sodium: 160mg,Carbohydrates: 6.

Atlantic Cod With Basil Walnut Sauce
Servings:4 | Cooking Time:x

Ingredients:
- 2 (6-ounce) Atlantic cod fillets
- 1/4 teaspoon kosher salt, divided
- 1/2 teaspoon freshly ground black pepper, divided
- Zest of 1 large lemon
- 3 tablespoons extra-virgin olive oil, divided
- 1/4 packed cup fresh basil leaves
- 1 tablespoon small walnut pieces

Directions:
1. Preheat oven to 400°F.
2. Place fish fillets in a 9" x 13" baking dish and sprinkle 1/8 teaspoon salt, 1/4 teaspoon pepper, and lemon zest over both sides of fish. Brush with 1 tablespoon olive oil.
3. Using a food processor, combine basil, walnuts, 1/8 teaspoon salt, and 1/4 teaspoon pepper. Process until it becomes a paste. With processor running, gradually add 2 tablespoons olive oil. Pat mixture evenly over fish.
4. Place baking dish in oven and bake for 13–17 minutes or until flesh is opaque in color. Serve with rice, spooning the juices from the pan over the fish and rice.

Nutrition Info:
- Calories: 176,Fat: 12g,Protein: 16g,Sodium: 194mg,Carbohydrates:2.

Rita's Linguine With Clam Sauce
Servings:4 | Cooking Time:x

Ingredients:
- 12 ounces gluten-free linguine
- 1 tablespoon olive oil
- 1 tablespoon garlic-infused olive oil
- 1/8 teaspoon wheat-free asafetida powder
- 2 tablespoons unsalted butter, divided
- 1/2 cup dry white wine
- 1 teaspoon dried oregano
- 2 dozen cherrystone clams, rinsed and scrubbed
- 1/4 cup coarsely chopped fresh flat-leaf parsley
- 1/2 teaspoon freshly ground black pepper

Directions:

1. Cook pasta until al dente according to package directions. Reserve 1/2 cup pasta water; drain pasta. Set aside.
2. While pasta cooks, heat oils over medium heat in a 5-quart saucepan. Add asafetida, 1 tablespoon butter, wine, and oregano and bring to a boil; cook 2 minutes.
3. Add clams; cover and simmer until clams open, about 10 minutes. If any clams have not opened, discard.
4. Add pasta to clams and stir 1 minute. Remove from heat and stir in 1 tablespoon butter, parsley, black pepper, and reserved pasta water; stir to combine. Serve immediately.

Nutrition Info:
- Calories: 456,Fat: 14g,Protein: 12g,Sodium: 14mg,Carbohydrates: 65.

Shrimp And Cheese Casserole

Servings:4 | Cooking Time:x

Ingredients:
- 3 tablespoons butter
- 1/8 teaspoon salt
- 1/8 teaspoon freshly ground black pepper
- 1/8 teaspoon wheat-free asafetida powder
- 1/4 cup dry white wine
- 10 ounces fresh spinach, chopped
- 1 (14.5-ounce) can diced tomatoes, drained
- 10 ounces medium shrimp, peeled and deveined
- 2 tablespoons olive oil
- 1/4 pound crumbled feta cheese
- 1/4 pound shredded mozzarella cheese

Directions:
1. Preheat oven to 350°F. Grease a 9" × 13" casserole dish.
2. In a large skillet, melt butter over medium-high heat; add salt, pepper, and asafetida and stir.
3. Add wine and spinach and cook 2–3 minutes.
4. Put spinach mixture into prepared casserole dish and layer in diced tomatoes. Place shrimp on top, drizzle with olive oil. Sprinkle with feta and mozzarella.
5. Bake 25 minutes or until cheese is bubbly and slightly brown.

Nutrition Info:
- Calories: 346,Fat: 22g,Protein: 27g,Sodium: 790mg,Carbohydrates: 8.

Creamy Halibut

Servings:4 | Cooking Time:x

Ingredients:
- 2 teaspoons sunflower oil
- 1 1/2 pounds halibut, cut into 4 portions
- 1/3 cup Basic Mayonnaise (see Chapter 13)
- 2 1/2 tablespoons lemon juice
- 2 1/4 tablespoons grated Parmesan cheese
- 1/8 teaspoon wheat-free asafetida powder
- 1 teaspoon Dijon mustard
- 1/2 teaspoon crushed red pepper flakes
- 2 tablespoons chopped fresh flat-leaf parsley

Directions:
1. Preheat oven to 400°F.
2. Heat oil in a large nonstick skillet over medium-high heat. Brown halibut on both sides, about 3 minutes each side.
3. Remove fish from skillet and place in a 9" × 13" ovenproof casserole dish. Bake 7 minutes.
4. While fish is baking, mix together remaining ingredients except parsley in a medium bowl.
5. Once fish is done baking, spoon mixture over fish and broil in oven 2 minutes. Garnish with parsley.

Nutrition Info:
- Calories: 358,Fat: 22g,Protein: 37g,Sodium: 267mg,Carbohydrates: 2.

Shrimp Puttanesca With Linguine

Servings:4 | Cooking Time:x

Ingredients:
- 1 pound gluten-free linguine
- 2 tablespoons olive oil
- 1 (24-ounce) can diced tomatoes
- 2 cups shredded kale
- 1/2 cup black olives
- 1/2 cup green olives
- 2 tablespoons capers, rinsed and drained
- 1 teaspoon red pepper flakes
- 1 pound large shrimp
- 1/2 cup crumbled feta cheese

Directions:
1. Cook pasta according to package directions. Drain and set aside.
2. Heat oil in a large skillet over medium heat. Stir in tomatoes, kale, black and green olives, capers, and red pepper flakes. Bring to a boil, then reduce heat to a simmer and cook 15 minutes.
3. Add pasta, shrimp, and cheese to sauce. Cook 3–5 minutes or until shrimp is cooked through.

Nutrition Info:
- Calories: 529,Fat: 18g,Protein: 42g,Sodium: 1,130mg,Carbohydrates: 98.

Cornmeal-crusted Tilapia

Servings:2 | Cooking Time:x

Ingredients:
- 1 pound tilapia
- 1/4 cup gluten-free bread crumbs
- 3/4 cup coarse cornmeal
- 2 tablespoons gluten-free all-purpose flour
- 1/2 teaspoon salt
- 1 teaspoon freshly ground black pepper
- 1/8 teaspoon wheat-free asafetida powder
- 1 large egg
- 1 tablespoon lactose-free milk
- 1 tablespoon sunflower oil

Directions:
1. Rinse and pat fish dry. Slice into 2 pieces.
2. In a large bowl, combine bread crumbs, cornmeal, flour, salt, pepper, and asafetida. In a small bowl, whisk together egg and milk.
3. Dip tilapia in egg mixture, tapping off any excess. Then dip both sides of fish in cornmeal mixture.
4. Heat oil in a 9" frying pan on medium-high heat. Pan-fry fish 3–5 minutes each side; fish should be opaque throughout and flaky.

Nutrition Info:
- Calories: 561, Fat: 13g, Protein: 50g, Sodium: 882mg, Carbohydrates: 58.

Salmon Noodle Casserole

Servings:8 | Cooking Time:x

Ingredients:
- 3 small sweet potatoes
- 1 pound gluten-free egg noodles
- 1/4 cup Sweet Barbecue Sauce (see recipe in Chapter 9)
- 1 (5-ounce) can salmon, drained and flaked with a fork
- 1 cup freshly grated Parmesan cheese, divided
- 2 slices gluten-free bread, toasted
- 1/2 cup shelled pecans
- 1 teaspoon sea salt, divided
- 1/2 teaspoon freshly ground pepper, divided
- 3/4 cup lactose-free whole milk
- 1/4 cup lactose-free plain low-fat yogurt
- 1 cup Vegetable Stock (see recipe in Chapter 8)
- 1 cup shredded fontina cheese
- 1 cup packed baby spinach leaves

Directions:
1. Preheat oven to 400°F. Poke a few holes in each sweet potato and place in a small baking dish. Bake sweet potatoes for 45 minutes. Remove from oven, slice open to cool, and set aside.
2. Cook noodles according to package directions to an al dente texture.
3. Heat barbecue sauce in a small skillet over medium heat. Add salmon and sauté very carefully for about 3 minutes until fully coated. Remove from heat.
4. In a food processor, add 1/2 cup Parmesan cheese, toast, pecans, 1/2 teaspoon salt, and 1/4 teaspoon pepper. Pulse to a bread-crumb consistency. Transfer to a medium bowl.
5. Once cool enough to handle, scoop inside flesh from sweet potatoes and transfer to food processor. Add milk, yogurt, stock, and remaining salt and pepper and process to combine.
6. Add fontina and remaining 1/2 cup Parmesan cheese and pulse until combined.
7. Transfer noodles to a 13" × 9" baking dish. Pour sweet potato mixture over noodles and stir to combine.
8. Tuck spinach leaves between the noodles. Dot top of casserole evenly with salmon mixture.
9. Sprinkle top of casserole evenly with bread-crumb mixture. Bake 20 minutes, or until cheese is melted and bubbling or browning. Let sit for 5 minutes, then serve.

Nutrition Info:
- Calories: 510, Fat: 19g, Protein: 25g, Sodium: 1,140mg, Carbohydrates: 61.

Light Tuna Casserole

Servings:8 | Cooking Time:x

Ingredients:
- 1 tablespoon butter
- 2 large carrots, peeled and diced
- 1/4 cup gluten-free all-purpose flour
- 1 1/2 cups chicken stock
- 1 1/2 cups lactose-free milk
- 1 cup frozen green beans, thawed
- 1 teaspoon dried oregano
- 1 teaspoon dried marjoram
- 1 teaspoon dried rosemary
- 1 teaspoon dried thyme
- 1/2 teaspoon salt
- 1/4 teaspoon freshly ground black pepper
- 3 (5-ounce) cans tuna in water, drained
- 8 ounces gluten-free egg noodles, cooked al dente
- 1/2 cup shredded sharp Cheddar cheese
- 1/2 cup shredded Colby cheese
- 2 tablespoons gluten-free panko bread crumbs

Directions:
1. Preheat oven to 400°F.
2. Melt butter in a large saucepan over medium-high heat. Add carrots, and sauté 5–7 minutes, or until soft. Stir in flour and cook 1 minute.
3. Whisk in stock, then stir in milk, green beans, oregano, marjoram, rosemary, thyme, salt, pepper, and tuna. Continue cooking, stirring occasionally, about 5 minutes.
4. Add sauce mixture to noodles and toss to combine. Stir in Cheddar and Colby cheese.
5. Pour noodles into a greased 9" × 13" baking pan. Sprinkle bread crumbs on top. Bake 18–20 minutes or until top is crispy and golden and filling is bubbling. Serve immediately.

Nutrition Info:
- Calories: 339, Fat: 11g, Protein: 23g, Sodium: 650mg, Carbohydrates: 35.

Salmon Cakes With Fresh Dill Sauce

Servings:8 | Cooking Time:x

Ingredients:
- 1 pound skinless wild-caught salmon fillet
- 3 scallions, chopped, green part only, divided
- 2 tablespoons lemon juice, divided
- 2 tablespoons Dijon mustard
- 1 teaspoon salt, divided
- 1/4 teaspoon freshly ground black pepper
- 1/4 cup gluten-free panko bread crumbs
- 1 tablespoon coconut oil
- 2 tablespoons fresh dill
- 7 ounces lactose-free sour cream

Directions:
1. In a food processor, pulse salmon, 2 scallions, 1 tablespoon lemon juice, mustard, 1/2 teaspoon salt, and pepper until coarsely chopped.
2. Mix in the bread crumbs and form into 8 patties.
3. Heat oil in a large nonstick skillet over medium heat. Cook patties until opaque throughout, about 2 minutes per side.
4. Dill sauce: In your food processor combine dill, sour cream, 1 tablespoon lemon juice, and 1/2 teaspoon salt. Pulse until blended. Dollop onto salmon cakes. Sprinkle on remaining scallions.

Nutrition Info:
- Calories: 160,Fat: 11g,Protein: 12g,Sodium: 409mg,Carbohydrates: 4.

Grilled Cod With Fresh Basil

Servings:4 | Cooking Time:x

Ingredients:
- 3 tablespoons extra-virgin olive oil
- Juice of 1 medium lemon
- 2 pounds cod fillet
- 1 garlic clove, peeled, slightly smashed
- 8 tablespoons butter (1 stick)
- 2 tablespoons chopped fresh basil
- 1 pinch ground red pepper

Directions:
1. Combine oil and lemon juice in a shallow dish. Add cod and turn to coat. Marinate for 30 minutes at room temperature.
2. Heat a charcoal or gas grill to 350ºF. Grill fish for 15 minutes or until cooked through, flipping once after 8 minutes.
3. When fish is on its second side, put garlic and butter in a small saucepan and cook over low heat for 5 minutes. Turn off heat, remove and discard the garlic, and add basil and ground red pepper.
4. Remove cod from grill and serve with basil sauce on the side.

Nutrition Info:
- Calories: 400,Fat: 25g,Protein: 40g,Sodium: 125mg,Carbohydrates: 1.

Seafood Risotto

Servings:6 | Cooking Time:x

Ingredients:
- 2 1/2 cups water
- 2 (8-ounce) bottles clam juice
- 6 tablespoons olive oil, divided
- 1 1/2 cups arborio rice
- 1/2 cup dry white wine
- 3/4 pound uncooked large shrimp, peeled, deveined, coarsely chopped
- 3/4 pound bay scallops
- 1/8 teaspoon wheat-free asafetida powder
- 1 tablespoon butter
- 1/2 cup grated Parmesan cheese
- 2 tablespoons finely chopped fresh Italian parsley

Directions:
1. Combine water and clam juice in a medium saucepan. Bring to simmer. Keep warm over low heat.
2. Heat 3 tablespoons oil in heavy, large saucepan over medium heat. Add rice; sauté 2 minutes.
3. Add wine; stir until liquid is absorbed, about 2 minutes. Add 1 cup clam juice mixture to rice. Simmer until liquid is absorbed, stirring often. Continue adding clam juice mixture 1/2 cup at a time, stirring often and simmering until liquid is absorbed before each addition. Simmer until rice is tender but still slightly firm in center and mixture is creamy, about 25 minutes.
4. Heat remaining 3 tablespoons oil in a separate heavy, large skillet over medium-high heat. Add shrimp, scallops, and asafetida. Sauté until shrimp and scallops are opaque in center, about 6 minutes.
5. Add seafood to rice. Stir and add butter; cook 4 minutes longer. Remove from heat and stir in Parmesan cheese. Transfer to serving bowl.
6. Garnish with chopped parsley and serve.

Nutrition Info:
- Calories: 514,Fat: 22g,Protein: 30g,Sodium: 478mg,Carbohydrates: 43.

Mediterranean Flaky Fish With Vegetables

Servings:4 | Cooking Time:x

Ingredients:
- 4 (3.5-ounce) skinless Atlantic cod fillets
- 1 cup grated zucchini
- 1/4 cup thinly sliced fresh basil, plus 4 whole basil leaves
- 20 cherry tomatoes, halved
- 10 black olives, sliced
- 1/4 teaspoon kosher salt
- 1/2 teaspoon freshly ground black pepper
- 4 tablespoons dry white wine, divided
- 4 tablespoons extra-virgin olive oil, divided

Directions:
1. Preheat oven to 400°F.
2. Make parchment pockets: Pull out a 17" × 11" piece of parchment paper. With one longer edge closest to you, fold in half from left to right. Using scissors, cut out a large heart shape. On a large cutting board or clean work surface, lay down parchment heart and place fish on one half of heart, leaving at least a 1½" border around fillet. Repeat with remaining fish fillets. Lay parchment hearts in a 9" × 13" baking dish.
3. In a medium bowl, combine zucchini, sliced basil, tomatoes, olives, salt, and pepper. Stir to combine.
4. Evenly distribute the vegetables over each fish fillet in the parchment hearts.
5. Take opposite side of each parchment heart and fold over, making both edges of heart line up. Starting at rounded end, crimp edges together tightly. Leave a few inches at pointed end unfolded. Grab pointed edge and tilt heart to pour in 1 tablespoon each of wine and oil. Finish by crimping edges and twisting pointed end around and under packet.
6. Bake until just cooked through, about 10–12 minutes. Poke a toothpick through parchment paper. Fish should be done if toothpick easily slides through fish. Carefully cut open packets (steam will escape). Garnish with whole basil leaves.

Nutrition Info:
- Calories: 246,Fat: 16g,Protein: 19g,Sodium: 304mg,Carbohydrates: 6.

Tilapia Piccata
Servings:6 | Cooking Time:x

Ingredients:
- ¼ cup dry white wine
- 3 tablespoons freshly squeezed lemon juice, preferably Meyer
- 1 teaspoon fresh lemon zest
- 2 tablespoons capers, rinsed, drained
- ¼ cup sweet rice flour, divided
- ½ teaspoon sea salt
- ¼ teaspoon freshly ground black pepper
- 4 (6-ounce) pieces tilapia fillets
- 1 tablespoon Garlic-Infused Oil (see recipe in Chapter 9)
- 1 teaspoon butter
- 1 tablespoon chopped fresh parsley

Directions:
1. In a small bowl, whisk wine, lemon juice, zest, and capers.
2. Reserve 1 teaspoon flour and set aside. Mix remaining flour with salt and pepper on a plate. Dip fish into flour.
3. Heat oil over medium heat in a large skillet. Add fish and cook 2–3 minutes per side. When fish is cooked through, remove from pan.
4. Add wine mixture and reserved flour to pan and cook 1 minute, whisking constantly. Remove from heat and stir in butter.
5. Top fish with the sauce, garnish with parsley, and serve immediately.

Nutrition Info:
- Calories: 168,Fat: 5g,Protein: 23g,Sodium: 342mg,Carbohydrates: 6.

Basic Baked Scallops
Servings:2 | Cooking Time:x

Ingredients:
- ¾ pound sea scallops
- 2 tablespoons lemon juice
- 2½ tablespoons unsalted butter, melted
- ¼ teaspoon sea salt
- ½ teaspoon freshly ground black pepper
- 2 tablespoons chopped fresh flat-leaf parsley
- ½ cup gluten-free bread crumbs
- ½ teaspoon smoked paprika
- 2 tablespoons olive oil

Directions:
1. Preheat oven to 425°F.
2. Toss together scallops, lemon juice, melted butter, salt, and pepper in a 2-quart baking dish.
3. In a medium bowl, combine parsley, bread crumbs, paprika, and olive oil. Sprinkle on top of scallops.
4. Bake 12–14 minutes or until scallops are heated through and bread crumbs are golden. Serve immediately.

Nutrition Info:
- Calories: 426,Fat: 30g,Protein: 17g,Sodium: 621mg,Carbohydrates: 23.

Grilled Halibut With Lemony Pesto
Servings:4 | Cooking Time:x

Ingredients:
- 1 tablespoon grapeseed oil
- 2 tablespoons freshly squeezed lemon juice, divided
- 2 teaspoons grated lemon zest, divided
- ½ teaspoon sea salt
- ¼ teaspoon freshly ground black pepper
- 4 (6-ounce) raw halibut steaks
- ½ cup Garden Pesto (see recipe in Chapter 9)

Directions:
1. Whisk oil, 1 tablespoon lemon juice, 1 teaspoon zest, salt, and pepper in a large bowl. Add halibut and marinate for 30 minutes.
2. Add pesto, remaining juice, and remaining zest to a food processor. Pulse just until combined.
3. Heat a charcoal grill, gas grill, or broiler to 350°F. Grill or broil steaks, about 6 minutes per side until fish is cooked through.
4. Top fish with the lemony pesto and serve immediately.

Nutrition Info:
- Calories: 356,Fat: 20g,Protein: 39g,Sodium: 675mg,Car-

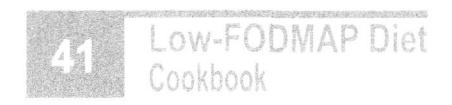

bohydrates: 3.

Baked Moroccan-style Halibut

Servings:4 | Cooking Time:x

Ingredients:
- 1 pint cherry tomatoes
- 1/4 cup pitted black olives
- 1/8 teaspoon wheat-free asafetida powder
- 1/2 teaspoon ground cumin
- 1/4 teaspoon ground cinnamon
- 1/4 teaspoon freshly ground black pepper
- 4 (6-ounce) fresh halibut fillets
- 2 tablespoons olive oil

Directions:
1. Preheat oven 450°F.
2. In a medium mixing bowl, stir together tomatoes, olives, asafetida, cumin, cinnamon, and black pepper.
3. Add halibut to a large baking dish. Sprinkle tomato mixture evenly over fish. Drizzle oil over fish.
4. Bake 10–15 minutes or until an instant-read thermometer inserted into the thickest fillet reads 145°F. Serve immediately.

Nutrition Info:
- Calories: 269,Fat: 12g,Protein: 36g,Sodium: 168mg,Carbohydrates: 4.

Poached Salmon With Tarragon Sauce

Servings:4 | Cooking Time:x

Ingredients:
- 1/2 cup Basic Mayonnaise (see Chapter 13)
- 1/2 cup lactose-free sour cream
- 2 teaspoons chopped fresh tarragon
- 1 tablespoon chopped green onion, green part only
- 1 tablespoon lemon juice
- 1/8 teaspoon sea salt, divided
- 1 teaspoon freshly ground black pepper, divided
- 1 3/4 cups dry white wine
- 2 cups water
- 2-pound salmon fillet with skin

Directions:
1. In a food processor combine mayonnaise, sour cream, tarragon, onion, lemon juice, 1/16 teaspoon salt, and 1/2 teaspoon pepper; purée until smooth. (Make 1 day ahead if desired; chill and cover.) If making sauce ahead of time, allow sauce to cool to room temperature before serving.
2. In a deep 12" skillet bring water and wine to a simmer, covered.
3. Cut salmon into 4 pieces and season with 1/16 teaspoon salt and 1/2 teaspoon pepper. Submerge salmon skin-side down in pot. Make sure there is enough water to cover salmon. Simmer about 8 minutes or until just cooked through. Do not overcook fish.
4. Using a slotted spatula to drain any excess water, transfer salmon to a platter or dish to cool. Once salmon is cool, remove skin. Let salmon cool to room temperature before serving. Spoon tarragon sauce over salmon.

Nutrition Info:
- Calories: 516,Fat: 25g,Protein: 45g,Sodium: 380mg,Carbohydrates: 11.

Cedar Planked Salmon

Servings:4 | Cooking Time:x

Ingredients:
- Cedar grilling plank
- 1 tablespoon demerara sugar
- 1 teaspoon freshly ground tricolored peppercorns
- 1/4 teaspoon sea salt
- 1/8 teaspoon pure vanilla extract
- 12-ounce raw salmon fillet

Directions:
1. Prepare cedar plank by soaking in warm water for at least 1 hour.
2. In a small bowl, mix sugar, peppercorns, salt, and vanilla. Rub all over salmon and transfer, skin-side down, to prepared plank.
3. Heat a charcoal grill, gas grill, or broiler to 350°F. Grill or broil salmon, skin-side down on plank, for 15 minutes.

Nutrition Info:
- Calories: 133,Fat: 5g,Protein: 17g,Sodium: 185mg,Carbohydrates: 4.

Glazed Salmon

Servings:4 | Cooking Time:x

Ingredients:
- 1/4 cup gluten-free tamari
- 1 tablespoon almond butter
- 1 tablespoon pure maple syrup
- 2 teaspoons rice vinegar
- 2 teaspoons sesame oil
- 1 teaspoon blackstrap molasses
- 1/8 teaspoon ground ginger
- 12-ounce fillet of salmon

Directions:
1. Make glaze: Mix all ingredients except salmon in a small saucepan.
2. Transfer 2 tablespoons glaze to a small bowl.
3. Heat a charcoal grill, gas grill, or broiler to 350°F. Grill or broil salmon, skin-side down, for 15 minutes, basting with the sauce in the small bowl.
4. While salmon is cooking, heat remaining glaze over medium-low heat for about 5 minutes to thicken.
5. When salmon is fully cooked, remove from heat, drizzle with heated glaze, and serve.

Nutrition Info:
- Calories: 190,Fat: 10g,Protein: 19g,Sodium: 955mg,Carbohydrates: 6.

Coconut-crusted Fish With Pineapple Relish

Servings:2 | Cooking Time:x

Ingredients:
- 1/2 cup shredded unsweetened coconut
- 1/2 cup gluten-free panko bread crumbs
- 1/2 teaspoon paprika
- 1 large egg
- 1 pound cod fillets
- 2 cups chopped pineapple
- 1/4 cup finely chopped red bell pepper
- 1 tablespoon fresh lemon juice
- 2 teaspoons palm sugar
- 1 finely chopped seeded jalapeño pepper
- 1/8 teaspoon salt

Directions:
1. Preheat oven to 400°F.
2. In a medium bowl, mix together coconut, bread crumbs, and paprika. In a separate small bowl whisk egg. Dredge fish fillets in egg, then coconut-panko mixture.
3. Place in a baking pan and bake 12–15 minutes or until firm.
4. Make pineapple relish by combining pineapple, bell pepper, lemon juice, sugar, and jalapeño pepper and then stirring in salt. Top fish with relish and serve.

Nutrition Info:
- Calories: 423,Fat: 11g,Protein: 46g,Sodium: 224mg,Carbohydrates: 36.

Grilled Swordfish With Pineapple Salsa

Servings:4 | Cooking Time:x

Ingredients:
- 2 tablespoons finely chopped cilantro
- 2 medium limes, juiced and zested
- 1 medium orange, juiced and zested
- 1/2 whole pineapple, cut into small chunks
- 1/4 teaspoon kosher salt
- 1/2 teaspoon freshly ground black pepper
- 4 (3.5-ounce) swordfish steaks, 1" thick
- 2 tablespoons olive oil

Directions:
1. In a medium bowl, combine cilantro, lime and orange juice and zest, and pineapple; set aside.
2. Set a gas grill to medium-high or heat a cast-iron skillet over medium-high heat. Mix salt and pepper together in a small bowl.
3. Brush swordfish with oil and sprinkle with salt and pepper.
4. Cook fish 5 minutes on one side and 3 minutes on other side.
5. Transfer swordfish to plates; top with pineapple salsa.

Nutrition Info:
- Calories: 267,Fat: 11g,Protein: 20g,Sodium: 238mg,Carbohydrates: 24.

Sole Meunière

Servings:2 | Cooking Time:x

Ingredients:
- 2 (4-ounce) boneless, skinless sole fillets
- 1/4 teaspoon kosher salt
- 1/4 teaspoon freshly ground black pepper
- 1/4 cup gluten-free all-purpose flour
- 4 tablespoons unsalted butter, divided
- 1 1/2 tablespoons finely chopped fresh flat-leaf parsley
- 1/2 teaspoon grated lemon zest
- Pulp 1/2 large lemon, seeds removed

Directions:
1. Season fillets on both sides with salt and pepper and lay on a plate. Place flour in a shallow bowl. Dredge fillets in flour, shaking off any excess.
2. Heat 2 tablespoons butter in a 12" skillet over medium-high heat. Place fillets in skillet and cook until browned on both sides and just cooked through, about 6 minutes.
3. Transfer fillets to plates; sprinkle with parsley.
4. Using a paper towel, carefully wipe skillet clean and return to heat. Add remaining butter, stir, and cook until it starts to brown. Add lemon zest and pulp; cook 3–4 minutes, then pour over fillets. Serve immediately.

Nutrition Info:
- Calories: 364,Fat: 25g,Protein: 23g,Sodium: 390mg,Carbohydrates: 12.

Citrusy Swordfish Skewers

Servings:4 | Cooking Time:x

Ingredients:
- 2 medium oranges, peeled
- 4 (4-ounce) swordfish steaks
- 2 tablespoons Garlic-Infused Oil (see recipe in Chapter 9)
- 1 tablespoon orange juice
- 1 teaspoon dried oregano
- 1/2 teaspoon sea salt

Directions:
1. Cut each orange into six equal parts. Cut swordfish into 2" cubes.
2. Combine oil, orange juice, oregano, and salt in a medium bowl. Whisk marinade; add fish and orange pieces. Toss to coat. Marinate for 60 minutes, tossing occasionally.
3. Skewer the swordfish and orange pieces in an alternating fish/fruit pattern.
4. Heat grill or broiler to medium. Grill or broil skewers for 15 minutes, turning once, until fish is cooked through. Serve immediately.

Nutrition Info:
- Calories: 230,Fat: 11g,Protein: 23g,Sodium: 395mg,Carbohydrates: 9.

Shrimp With Cherry Tomatoes

Servings:4 | Cooking Time:x

Ingredients:
- 1 pound gluten-free spaghetti
- 2 medium zucchini, trimmed
- 1 pound carrots, peeled
- 3 tablespoons extra-virgin olive oil, divided
- 1 pint cherry tomatoes, halved
- 3 tablespoons butter
- 3 tablespoons white wine
- Juice of 1 medium lemon
- 2 tablespoons chopped fresh basil
- 2 cloves garlic, peeled and slightly crushed
- 1 1/2 pounds peeled and deveined shrimp
- 1/8 teaspoon sea salt
- 1/8 teaspoon freshly ground black pepper

Directions:
1. Cook spaghetti according to package directions.
2. With vegetable peeler, peel zucchini and carrots into long strips. Heat 1 tablespoon of oil in a large skillet over medium heat. Add vegetables and sauté until soft, approximately 5–8 minutes, stirring frequently. Transfer to a bowl and keep warm. Wipe the skillet clean with a paper towel.
3. In a medium skillet, combine tomatoes, butter, wine, lemon juice, and basil. Cook over low heat for 10 minutes, stirring occasionally, then keep warm.
4. While tomatoes are cooking, heat the remaining 2 tablespoons of oil in the large skillet over medium heat. Add garlic and sauté until just starting to brown, about 5 minutes. Remove garlic and add shrimp to oil. Sauté shrimp until cooked through, approximately 8 minutes, stirring frequently. Season with salt and pepper.
5. To serve, place spaghetti on a serving platter and top with vegetable mixture, shrimp, and tomato mixture.

Nutrition Info:
- Calories: 848,Fat: 24g,Protein: 52g,Sodium: 420mg,Carbohydrates: 103.

Salmon With Herbs

Servings:2 | Cooking Time:x

Ingredients:
- 1 pound salmon fillets
- 1/4 teaspoon salt
- 1/2 teaspoon freshly ground black pepper
- 1/4 cup plus 2 tablespoons olive oil
- 1/4 cup chopped fresh dill
- 2 tablespoons roughly chopped fresh rosemary
- 1/4 cup fresh flat-leaf parsley leaves
- 2 tablespoons fresh thyme leaves
- 2 tablespoons lemon juice

Directions:
1. Preheat oven to 250°F.
2. Coat a 9" × 13" casserole dish with cooking spray. Lay salmon skin-side down and sprinkle with salt and pepper.
3. Blend 1/4 cup plus 2 tablespoons olive oil with dill, rosemary, parsley, thyme, and lemon juice in a small food processor. Use a spatula or your hands to pat the herb paste over the salmon.
4. Bake 22–28 minutes depending on thickness of salmon. Insert tines of a fork into thickest part of fillet and gently pull. If fish flakes easily, it is done.
5. Slide a spatula under fish and set on a cutting board. Cut into equal pieces and serve.

Nutrition Info:
- Calories: 588,Fat: 44g,Protein: 45g,Sodium: 403mg,Carbohydrates: 3.

Feta Crab Cakes

Servings:4 | Cooking Time:x

Ingredients:
- 5 slices gluten-free bread, toasted
- 1/2 teaspoon sea salt
- 1/8 teaspoon freshly ground black pepper
- 12 ounces lump cooked crabmeat
- 1/2 cup crumbled feta cheese
- 1/2 teaspoon dried basil
- 1/2 teaspoon dried oregano
- 1/2 teaspoon dried marjoram
- 1/2 teaspoon dried thyme
- 1 tablespoon lactose-free plain low-fat yogurt
- 1 large egg, beaten, divided

Directions:
1. Preheat oven to 400°F. Line a baking sheet with parchment paper and brush with safflower oil.
2. Add toast, salt, and pepper to a food processor. Pulse until fine bread crumbs form.
3. In a large bowl, combine 1/3 cup bread crumbs, crabmeat, feta, basil, oregano, marjoram, thyme, yogurt, and 1 tablespoon beaten egg. Stir well to combine.
4. Place remaining beaten egg in a bowl. Place remaining bread crumbs in a separate shallow bowl. Create 8 equal round balls of crab mixture. Working with one ball at a time, flatten to a 1/2" disc, then coat in egg, followed by bread crumbs. Transfer to baking sheet.
5. Bake 10 minutes, then carefully turn each cake over and bake 10 minutes more.

Nutrition Info:
- Calories: 270,Fat: 7g,Protein: 26g,Sodium: 1,065mg,Carbohydrates: 24.

Maple-glazed Salmon

Servings:2 | Cooking Time:x

Ingredients:
- 2 tablespoons toasted sesame seeds
- 3 tablespoons maple syrup
- 3 tablespoons sesame oil
- 1/4 cup gluten-free soy sauce (tamari)
- 1/8 teaspoon freshly ground black pepper
- 1/8 teaspoon wheat-free asafetida powder
- 2 (6-ounce) wild salmon fillets
- 1 tablespoon thinly sliced fresh gingerroot
- 2 scallions, chopped, green part only

Directions:
1. To toast sesame seeds, use a small dry skillet and place over medium heat. Toast 3–5 minutes or until lightly browned, stirring occasionally. Set aside on a plate.
2. In a large, shallow dish, whisk maple syrup, sesame oil, tamari, pepper, and asafetida. Once evenly combined, add salmon to mixture and using tongs, turn fish to evenly coat every side. Place ginger slices on top of salmon. Cover and refrigerate at least 2 hours. If possible, refrigerate up to 24 hours so more of the flavors marinate throughout the fish.
3. Preheat oven to 450°F.
4. Remove salmon from refrigerator and using tongs, coat both sides of fish with toasted sesame seeds. Place salmon in a 9" × 13" baking dish and cook 10–12 minutes or until salmon is opaque in center. An instant-read thermometer should register 145°F in thickest part of fillet.
5. Transfer to plates and garnish with scallions.

Nutrition Info:
- Calories: 573,Fat: 35g,Protein: 37g,Sodium: 1,876mg,-Carbohydrates: 26.

Fish And Chips

Servings:4 | Cooking Time:x

Ingredients:
- 1/4 cup millet
- 1/4 cup chopped pecans
- 2 tablespoons cornmeal
- 1 1/2 teaspoons sea salt, divided
- 1/8 teaspoon ground red pepper
- 4 small red potatoes, thinly sliced
- 1 tablespoon extra-virgin olive oil
- 1/2 cup lactose-free 2% milk
- 2 tablespoons light sour cream
- 12 ounces tilapia fillets

Directions:
1. In a medium bowl, cover millet with boiling water and soak for 30 minutes.
2. Preheat oven to 400°F. Line 2 baking sheets with parchment paper.
3. Drain millet completely and spread on one baking sheet. Add pecans to second baking sheet. Roast millet and pecans for 10 minutes, tossing halfway through.
4. Process pecans in a food processor until finely ground. Transfer to a medium shallow dish; toss with millet, cornmeal, 1/2 teaspoon salt, and red pepper.
5. Toss potato slices in oil and 1 teaspoon salt. Re-line one baking sheet and scatter it with potatoes. Roast in oven for 30 minutes or until brown and crisp.
6. In another shallow dish, whisk together milk and sour cream.
7. Re-line the second baking sheet and coat with cooking spray. Working with one piece at a time, dip tilapia in milk mixture and then carefully coat both sides in millet mixture. Transfer to baking sheet.
8. Bake for 15 minutes or until fish is cooked through. Serve with the potato chips.

Nutrition Info:
- Calories: 360,Fat: 12g,Protein: 24g,Sodium: 955mg,Carbohydrates: 42.

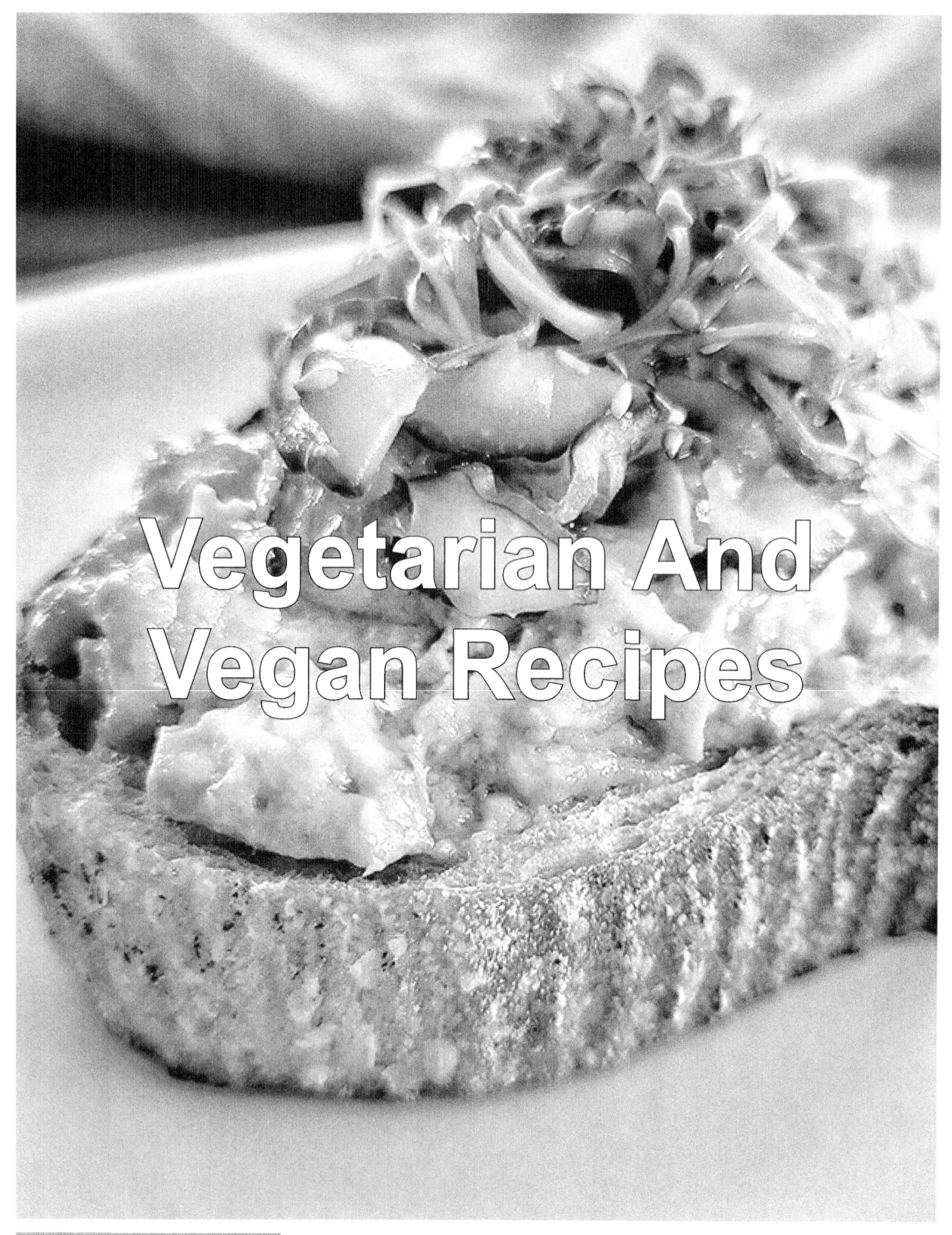

Vegetarian And Vegan Recipes

Vegetarian And Vegan Recipes

Tempeh Tacos
Servings:4 | Cooking Time:x

Ingredients:
- 1 (8-ounce) package tempeh
- 2 small vine-ripe tomatoes, chopped
- 1 teaspoon chili powder
- 1/2 teaspoon ground cumin
- 3 tablespoons lime juice, divided
- 2–4 tablespoons water
- 1 1/2 tablespoons coconut oil, divided
- 1/2 medium green bell pepper, seeded and diced
- 2 cups common (green) cabbage, diced
- 8 (6") soft corn tortillas, warmed
- 1 1/2 cups Fiesta Salsa (see recipe in Chapter 13)
- 1/2 medium avocado, cut into eighths

Directions:
1. Crumble tempeh into a large mixing bowl. Add tomatoes, chili powder, cumin, and 1 tablespoon lime juice. Stir in 1 tablespoon water and mix again. If tempeh mixture seems a little dry, add more water. Set aside.
2. Heat 1 tablespoon oil in large skillet over medium-high heat. Add bell pepper and cabbage. Cook for 10–12 minutes, stirring occasionally.
3. Add tempeh mixture and cook 8–10 minutes, stirring frequently. Halfway through cooking, add 1 tablespoon lime juice, 1 tablespoon water, and 1/2 tablespoon coconut oil. Add 2 more tablespoons of water and 1 tablespoon lime juice toward end of cooking. Stir again. Remove from heat. Mixture should be moist. Add more water if necessary.
4. Fill tortillas with tempeh mixture, salsa, and cabbage, and top with avocado.

Nutrition Info:
- Calories: 472,Fat: 24g,Protein: 19g,Sodium: 992mg,Carbohydrates: 52.

Tofu And Red Bell Pepper Quinoa
Servings:4 | Cooking Time: 21 Minutes

Ingredients:
- Rest: 5 minutes
- 2 tablespoons Garlic Oil
- 1 red bell pepper, chopped
- 6 ounces firm tofu, chopped
- 1 cup quinoa, rinsed well
- 2 cups Low-FODMAP Vegetable Broth
- 1 teaspoon dried thyme
- 1/2 teaspoon sea salt
- 1/4 teaspoon freshly ground black pepper

Directions:
1. In a large saucepan over medium-high heat, heat the garlic oil until it shimmers.
2. Add the bell pepper and the tofu. Cook for about 5 minutes, stirring, until the pepper is soft.
3. Add the quinoa. Cook for 1 minute, stirring.
4. Add the broth, thyme, salt, and pepper. Bring to a boil. Reduce the heat to medium and simmer for 15 minutes.
5. Turn off the heat. Cover the pot and let it sit for 5 minutes more.
6. Fluff with a fork.

Nutrition Info:
- Calories:276; Total Fat: 12g; Saturated Fat: 2g; Carbohydrates: 31g; Fiber: 4g; Sodium: 624mg; Protein: 12g

Vegan Noodles With Gingered Coconut Sauce
Servings:4 | Cooking Time: 10 Minutes

Ingredients:
- 1 tablespoon Garlic Oil (here)
- 2 1/2 tablespoons minced fresh ginger
- 1 (15-ounce) can light coconut milk
- 2 teaspoons sugar
- 2 teaspoons lemon juice
- 1 teaspoon salt
- 1/2 teaspoon freshly ground black pepper
- Red pepper flakes, to taste
- 1 bunch of Swiss chard leaves, thick center stems removed, leaves julienned
- 2 cups baby spinach
- 1 (16-ounce) package gluten-free spaghetti, cooked al dente according to package directions and drained
- 2 tablespoons chopped fresh basil

Directions:
1. Heat the Garlic Oil in a large sauté pan over medium heat. Add the ginger and cook, stirring, for about 3 minutes. Stir in the coconut milk, sugar, lemon juice, salt, pepper, and red pepper flakes and bring just to a boil. Reduce the heat to medium low and add the chard and spinach to the simmering sauce. Cook, stirring occasionally, until the greens are completely wilted, about 5 minutes.
2. Transfer the sauce mixture to a blender and purée, or transfer it to a bowl and purée it using an immersion blender.
3. Return the puréed sauce to the pan and bring it back to a simmer over medium heat. Add the prepared noodles and cook, stirring, until heated through, about 2 to 3 minutes. Serve immediately, garnished with basil.

Nutrition Info:
- Calories: 569; Protein: 11g; Total Fat: 15g; Saturated Fat: 1g; Carbohydrates: 99g; Fiber: 8g; Sodium: 908mg;

Roasted-veggie Gyros With Tzatziki Sauce

Servings:4 | Cooking Time: 35 Minutes

Ingredients:
- FOR THE ROASTED VEGETABLES
- 1 large zucchini, chopped into half moons
- 1 large yellow squash, chopped into half moons
- 1 large eggplant, cut into 1-inch cubes
- 1 cup cherry tomatoes, halved
- ¼ cup olive oil
- 1 tablespoon chopped fresh oregano
- 1½ teaspoons salt
- ¾ teaspoon freshly ground black pepper
- FOR THE SAUCE
- 1 medium cucumber, peeled, seeded, coarsely grated and squeezed in a clean dish towel to remove excess moisture
- 8 ounces plain lactose-free yogurt
- 1 tablespoon Garlic Oil (here)
- 1 tablespoon white-wine vinegar
- 1 tablespoon chopped fresh dill
- 1 tablespoon lemon juice
- TO SERVE
- 4 gluten-free pita pockets or gluten-free naan
- 4 large lettuce leaves

Directions:
1. Preheat the oven to 425°F.
2. On a large, rimmed baking sheet, toss the zucchini, yellow squash, eggplant, and cherry tomatoes together with the olive oil, oregano, salt, and pepper. Spread the vegetables out in an even layer and roast in the preheated oven for about 35 minutes, until they are soft and browned.
3. While the vegetables are roasting, make the sauce. In a medium bowl, combine the cucumber, yogurt, Garlic Oil, vinegar, dill, and lemon juice, and stir to combine. Refrigerate, covered, until ready to serve.
4. Wrap the pitas in foil and heat in the oven (you can place them in the oven along with the vegetables while they're roasting) for about 10 minutes.
5. To serve, fill each pita with the roasted vegetables, top with a dollop of the tzatziki sauce, and garnish each with a lettuce leaf. Serve immediately.

Nutrition Info:
- Calories: 342; Protein: 14g; Total Fat: 15g; Saturated Fat: 2g; Carbohydrates: 46g; Fiber: 12g; Sodium: 1023mg;

Stuffed Zucchini Boats

Servings:4 | Cooking Time: 40 Minutes

Ingredients:
- 4 medium zucchini, halved lengthwise with the middles scooped out, chopped, and reserved
- 2 cups cooked brown rice
- ½ cup canned crushed tomatoes, drained
- ½ cup grated Parmesan cheese
- ¼ cup chopped fresh basil leaves
- ½ teaspoon sea salt
- ⅛ teaspoon freshly ground black pepper

Directions:
1. Preheat the oven to 400°F.
2. Place the zucchini halves on a rimmed baking sheet, cut-side up.
3. In a medium bowl, stir together the brown rice, reserved chopped zucchini, tomatoes, Parmesan cheese, basil, salt, and pepper. Spoon the mixture into the zucchini boats.
4. Bake for 40 to 45 minutes, until the zucchini are soft.

Nutrition Info:
- Calories:262; Total Fat: 5g; Saturated Fat: 2g; Carbohydrates: 46g; Fiber: 5g; Sodium: 447mg; Protein: 11g

Cheese Strata

Servings:4 | Cooking Time: 30 Minutes

Ingredients:
- Nonstick cooking spray
- 3 eggs, beaten
- 1 cup unsweetened almond milk
- ½ teaspoon sea salt
- ⅛ teaspoon freshly ground black pepper
- 5 slices gluten-free sandwich bread, crusts removed, cut into cubes
- ¾ cup grated Monterey Jack cheese

Directions:
1. Preheat the oven to 350°F.
2. Spray a 9-by-5-inch loaf pan with nonstick cooking spray.
3. In a medium bowl, whisk together the eggs, almond milk, salt, and pepper.
4. Fold in the bread until it is coated with the egg mixture.
5. Fold in the cheese.
6. Pour the mixture into the prepared dish and bake for 30 to 35 minutes, until set.

Nutrition Info:
- Calories:402; Total Fat: 29g; Saturated Fat: 18g; Carbohydrates: 28g; Fiber: 6g; Sodium: 628mg; Protein: 12g

Mac 'n' Cheeze

Servings: 4 | Cooking Time: x

Ingredients:
- 1 pound brown rice pasta noodles
- 3 tablespoons nutritional yeast
- 1/2 teaspoon sea salt, divided
- 1/4 cup coconut oil
- 1/4 cup sweet rice flour
- 2 3/4 cups unsweetened almond milk
- 1 teaspoon rice wine vinegar
- 1/2 cup dairy-free cheese shreds
- 1/4 teaspoon freshly ground black pepper
- 1 teaspoon paprika

Directions:

1. Bring a large pot of salted water to a rolling boil and cook pasta until al dente according to package directions. Drain and set aside.
2. In a small bowl, combine yeast and 1/4 teaspoon sea salt. Set aside.
3. In a large skillet, heat coconut oil over medium-low heat. Whisk in flour and continue whisking constantly 3–5 minutes or until flour smells toasty but hasn't browned.
4. In a steady stream, whisk in almond milk, stirring constantly. Add yeast mixture and vinegar. Cook 3 minutes or until slightly thickened.
5. Add cheese shreds and mix until well incorporated.
6. Add pasta and toss with sauce, black pepper, and remaining salt. Cook 1–2 minutes more to reheat pasta. Sprinkle on paprika. Serve immediately.

Nutrition Info:
- Calories: 574, Fat: 16g, Protein: 13g, Sodium: 646mg, Carbohydrates: 91.

Kale-pesto Soba Noodles

Servings: 4 | Cooking Time: 10 Minutes

Ingredients:
- 1 (10-ounce) package gluten-free soba noodles
- 4 cups kale, removed from stems and roughly chopped
- Zest and juice of 1 lemon
- 1 cup pine nuts
- 3/4 cup grated Parmesan cheese, plus more for serving
- 3/4 cup olive oil
- 2 tablespoons Garlic Oil (here)
- 3/4 teaspoon salt
- 1/2 teaspoon freshly ground black pepper

Directions:

1. Cook the soba noodles according to the instructions on the package.
2. While the noodles are cooking, prepare the pesto. In a food processor, combine the kale, lemon zest and juice, pine nuts, and cheese, and pulse until the kale is finely chopped. With the processor running, slowly add the olive oil in a thin stream, and continue to process to a smooth purée. Add the Garlic Oil, salt, and pepper, and pulse to combine.
3. When the noodles are finished cooking, drain them and immediately toss them with the pesto. Serve immediately, garnished with additional cheese, if desired.

Nutrition Info:
- Calories: 922; Protein: 26g; Total Fat: 68g; Saturated Fat: 11g; Carbohydrates: 67g; Fiber: 4g; Sodium: 1293mg;

Curried Squash Soup With Coconut Milk

Servings: 4 | Cooking Time: 15 Minutes

Ingredients:
- 1 tablespoon coconut oil
- 1 tablespoon Garlic Oil (here)
- 1 tablespoon minced fresh ginger
- 8 pattypan squash, diced
- 2 medium zucchini, diced
- 1 teaspoon gluten-free, onion- and garlic-free curry powder
- 1 teaspoon salt
- 3/4 teaspoon ground coriander
- 1/2 teaspoon ground cumin
- 1/4 teaspoon ground cloves
- 1/4 teaspoon cayenne
- 4 cups homemade (onion- and garlic-free) vegetable broth
- 1/2 cup light coconut milk
- 1 cup pure pumpkin purée
- 2 tablespoons chopped fresh cilantro, for garnish

Directions:

1. Heat the coconut oil and Garlic Oil in a stockpot over medium-high heat. Add the ginger and cook for 1 minute. Add the pattypan squash and zucchini, and cook, stirring frequently, until the squash softens, about 3 minutes. Stir in the curry powder, salt, coriander, cumin, cloves, and cayenne, and cook, stirring, for 1 minute more. Add the broth, coconut milk, and pumpkin purée, and bring to a boil. Reduce the heat to low and simmer for about 10 minutes.
2. Purée the soup either in a blender in batches or in the pot using an immersion blender. Return to the heat if needed and heat through.
3. Serve hot, garnished with cilantro.

Nutrition Info:
- Calories: 155; Protein: 3g; Total Fat: 10g; Saturated Fat: 4g; Carbohydrates: 17g; Fiber: 4g; Sodium: 638mg;

Polenta With Roasted Vegetables And Spicy Tomato Sauce

Servings:4 | Cooking Time: 60 Minutes

Ingredients:
- FOR THE POLENTA
- Oil for preparing the baking sheet
- 4 cups water
- 1 teaspoon salt
- 1 cup uncooked polenta
- 2 tablespoons butter or nondairy butter substitute (optional)
- FOR THE VEGETABLES
- 2 medium red bell peppers, seeded and cut into ¼-inch-thick rings
- 2 cups assorted grape tomatoes
- 8 pieces oil-packed sun-dried tomatoes, julienned
- 2 tablespoons olive oil
- 1 teaspoon salt
- 1 teaspoon gluten-free, onion- and garlic-free chili powder
- 4 ounces crumbled queso fresco or feta cheese (optional)
- FOR THE SAUCE
- 2 jalapeño chiles, seeded and diced
- 1 tablespoon Garlic Oil (here)
- 1 teaspoon salt
- 1 (14½-ounce) can onion- and garlic-free diced tomatoes, preferably fire-roasted
- 2 tablespoons chopped fresh flat-leafed parsley

Directions:
1. Preheat the oven to 475°F.
2. Oil a large, rimmed baking sheet.
3. To make the polenta, combine the water and salt in a large saucepan, and bring to a boil over medium-high heat. While whisking continuously, slowly add the polenta. Reduce the heat to low and cook, whisking continuously, until the polenta becomes thick. Cover the saucepan and cook for about 30 minutes, stirring every once in a while, until the polenta is creamy and no grittiness remains. Just before serving, stir in the butter, if using.
4. In a large bowl, toss the bell peppers, grape tomatoes, and sun-dried tomatoes with the olive oil. Spread the vegetables on the baking sheet in a single layer. Sprinkle with the salt and chili powder. Roast in the preheated oven, stirring once or twice, until the vegetables are tender and starting to brown, for about 25 minutes.
5. Meanwhile, make the sauce. In a blender, combine the chiles, Garlic Oil, and salt, and blend until smooth. Add the tomatoes and pulse to a chunky, smooth texture. Transfer the mixture to a small saucepan and heat over medium heat. Simmer until the sauce is thickened, for about 6 minutes.
6. To serve, spoon some of the polenta into each of 4 serving bowls. Top with some of the roasted vegetables and spoon some of the warm sauce over the top. Sprinkle the cheese on top, if using. Garnish with parsley and serve immediately.

Nutrition Info:
- Calories: 457; Protein: 12g; Total Fat: 24g; Saturated Fat: 10g; Carbohydrates: 53g; Fiber: 8g; Sodium: 2135mg;

Coconut-curry Tofu With Vegetables

Servings:4 | Cooking Time: 25 Minutes

Ingredients:
- FOR THE SAUCE
- 1 cup canned coconut milk
- 2 tablespoons chopped fresh cilantro
- 1 tablespoon gluten-free, onion- and garlic-free curry powder
- 1 teaspoon brown sugar
- 1 teaspoon salt
- FOR THE TOFU AND VEGETABLES
- 1 tablespoon grapeseed oil
- 14 ounces extra-firm tofu, drained and cut into cubes
- 1 red bell pepper, sliced
- 1 zucchini, halved lengthwise and sliced
- 2 cups broccoli florets
- 1 bunch baby bok choy, cut into 2-inch pieces

Directions:
1. To make the sauce, in a small bowl, stir together the coconut milk, cilantro, curry powder, brown sugar, and salt.
2. To prepare the tofu and vegetables, heat the oil in a large skillet over high heat. Arrange the tofu in the pan in a single layer and cook, without stirring, for about 5 minutes, until it begins to brown on the bottom. Scrape the tofu from the pan with a spatula and continue to cook, stirring occasionally, until it is golden brown all over, for about 7 more minutes.
3. Add the bell pepper, zucchini, broccoli, and bok choy to the pan, along with the sauce mixture, and continue to cook, stirring, for about 8 to 10 minutes, until the vegetables are tender. Serve immediately.

Nutrition Info:
- Calories: 321; Protein: 16g; Total Fat: 25g; Saturated Fat: 14g; Carbohydrates: 17g; Fiber: 6g; Sodium: 756mg;

Zucchini Pizza Bites

Servings:4 | Cooking Time: 15 Minutes

Ingredients:
- 2 medium zucchini, cut into ¼-inch-thick slices
- 1 cup tomato sauce
- 2 tablespoons Garlic Oil
- 2 teaspoons dried Italian seasoning
- ½ teaspoon sea salt
- 1 cup grated mozzarella cheese

Directions:
1. Preheat the oven to 350°F.
2. Line two rimmed baking sheets with parchment paper. Arrange the zucchini slices in a single layer on the prepared sheets.

3. In a small bowl, whisk the tomato sauce, garlic oil, Italian seasoning, and salt. Spread the sauce on the zucchini slices.
4. Top with the cheese.
5. Bake for about 15 minutes, until the zucchini is soft and the cheese melts.

Nutrition Info:
- Calories:124; Total Fat: 6g; Saturated Fat: 3g; Carbohydrates: 9g; Fiber: 2g; Sodium: 736mg; Protein: 10g

Vegetable Stir-fry

Servings:4 | Cooking Time: 10 Minutes

Ingredients:
- 2 tablespoons Garlic Oil
- 2⅔ cups chopped firm tofu
- 8 scallions, green parts only, chopped
- 2 cups broccoli florets
- ½ cup Stir-Fry Sauce

Directions:
1. In a large skillet over medium-high heat, heat the garlic oil until it shimmers.
2. Add the tofu, scallions, and broccoli. Cook for about 7 minutes, stirring frequently, until the broccoli is crisp-tender.
3. Stir in the stir-fry sauce. Cook for about 3 minutes, stirring, until it thickens.

Nutrition Info:
- Calories:231; Total Fat: 14g; Saturated Fat: 3g; Carbohydrates: 14g; Fiber: 4g; Sodium: 426mg; Protein: 16g

Pasta With Tomato And Lentil Sauce

Servings:4 | Cooking Time: 10 Minutes

Ingredients:
- 2 tablespoons Garlic Oil
- 6 scallions, green parts only, chopped
- 2 cups canned lentils, drained
- 1½ cups canned crushed tomatoes, undrained
- 1 tablespoon dried Italian seasoning
- ½ teaspoon sea salt
- Pinch red pepper flakes
- ¼ cup chopped fresh basil leaves
- 8 ounces gluten-free pasta (any shape), cooked according to the package directions, drained

Directions:
1. In a large skillet over medium-high heat, heat the garlic oil until it shimmers.
2. Add the scallions and cook for 3 minutes.
3. Stir in the lentils, tomatoes, Italian seasoning, salt, and red pepper flakes. Simmer for 5 minutes, stirring.
4. Stir in the basil.
5. Add the hot pasta and toss to coat.

Nutrition Info:
- Calories:426; Total Fat: 3g; Saturated Fat: 0g; Carbohydrates: 73g; Fiber: 34g; Sodium: 461mg; Protein: 28g

Vegan Pad Thai

Servings:2 | Cooking Time:x

Ingredients:
- 2½ cups water, divided
- 1 (10-ounce) package rice noodles or ramen-style noodles
- 2 tablespoons peanut butter
- Juice of 2 medium limes
- 3 tablespoons palm sugar
- 1 chili (about 4" long), chopped and seeded
- 4 tablespoons gluten-free soy sauce (tamari), divided
- 2 tablespoons garlic-infused olive oil
- 1/2 (12-ounce package) extra-firm tofu, drained and cut into cubes
- 1 medium head broccoli, florets chopped small
- 2 cups bean sprouts
- 1 large scallion, green part only
- 2 tablespoons chopped unsalted peanuts

Directions:
1. Bring 1 1/2 cups water to boil in a medium pot and submerge noodles to soak. Turn off heat.
2. In a small bowl, whisk together peanut butter, lime juice, sugar, chili, 3 tablespoons soy sauce, and 1 cup water.
3. In a large frying pan, heat oil on medium and add tofu. Drizzle 1 tablespoon soy sauce over tofu and sauté until golden brown. Add broccoli and bean sprouts. Cook 4–5 minutes.
4. Drain noodles. Add peanut butter mixture and stir well. Add to tofu and cook through, about 5 minutes.
5. Garnish with scallions and peanuts. Serve immediately.

Nutrition Info:
- Calories: 454,Fat: 13g,Protein: 16g,Sodium: 920mg,Carbohydrates: 73.

Collard Green Wraps With Thai Peanut Dressing

Servings:3 | Cooking Time:x

Ingredients:
- 1/4 teaspoon salt
- 2 teaspoons lemon juice
- 6 large collard green leaves
- 9 ounces semi-firm tofu
- 2/3 cup bean sprouts
- 2 medium carrots, peeled and julienned
- 1 medium cucumber, peeled and julienned
- 2 tablespoons chopped fresh cilantro leaves
- 1/2 small avocado
- Thai Peanut Dressing (see Chapter 13)

Directions:
1. Set a wide saucepan over high heat. Fill with 3" of water. Add salt and lemon juice. Bring water to a simmer and reduce heat to medium. Place 1 collard green leaf at a time in water 35–45 seconds. When leaves are done, they should turn a bright-colored green. When done with each leaf, re-

move from water and place on a plate with paper towels to cool.

2. Place 1 1/2 ounces tofu toward top of each collard green leaf. Top each with an equal amount sprouts, carrots, cucumber, and cilantro. Cut out three (1/8) portions of avocado and place over vegetables. Drizzle Thai peanut dressing over vegetables.

3. Roll up wraps like you would a burrito, tucking in sides as you roll. Slice rolls in half and serve.

Nutrition Info:
- Calories: 255, Fat: 13g, Protein: 14g, Sodium: 713mg, Carbohydrates: 27.

Pineapple Fried Rice

Servings: 4 | Cooking Time: 10 Minutes

Ingredients:
- 2 tablespoons Garlic Oil
- 6 scallions, green parts only, finely chopped
- ½ cup canned water chestnuts, drained
- 1 tablespoon peeled and grated fresh ginger
- 3 cups cooked brown rice
- 2 cups canned pineapple (in juice), drained, ¼ cup juice reserved
- 2 tablespoons gluten-free soy sauce
- ¼ cup chopped fresh cilantro leaves

Directions:
1. In a large skillet over medium-high heat, heat the garlic oil until it shimmers.
2. Add the scallions, water chestnuts, and ginger. Cook for 5 minutes, stirring.
3. Add the brown rice, pineapple, reserved pineapple juice, and soy sauce. Cook for 5 minutes, stirring, until the rice is warmed through.
4. Stir in the cilantro.

Nutrition Info:
- Calories: 413; Total Fat: 9g; Saturated Fat: 1g; Carbohydrates: 77g; Fiber: 4g; Sodium: 396mg; Protein: 7g

Tempeh Enchiladas With Red Chili Sauce

Servings: 4 | Cooking Time: 60 Minutes

Ingredients:
- FOR THE SAUCE
- 2 tablespoons grapeseed oil
- 2 tablespoons gluten-free all-purpose flour
- 1 tablespoon Garlic Oil (here)
- ¼ cup gluten-free, onion- and garlic-free chili powder
- ½ teaspoon salt
- ¼ teaspoon ground cumin
- 1 tablespoon minced fresh oregano
- 2 cups homemade (onion- and garlic-free) vegetable broth
- FOR THE ENCHILADAS
- 12 ounces crumbled tempeh
- 2 cups canned corn kernels
- 1 (4-ounce) can diced green chiles
- 10 small corn tortillas
- 1½ cups shredded sharp white cheddar cheese (optional)

Directions:
1. To make the sauce, heat the grapeseed oil in a small saucepan over medium-high heat. Whisk in the flour and cook, stirring, for 1 minute. Stir in the Garlic Oil, chili powder, salt, cumin, and oregano. While stirring constantly, gradually add the broth. Bring to a boil, then reduce the heat to low and simmer, stirring occasionally, for 10 to 15 minutes, until the sauce has thickened. Transfer the sauce to a wide, shallow bowl.
2. In a bowl, stir together the crumbled tempeh, corn, and green chiles.
3. To make the enchiladas, spoon about ⅓ cup of the sauce into a 9-by-13-inch baking dish and spread it out over the bottom of the dish. Wrap the tortillas in a clean dish towel and heat them in the microwave on high for about 30 seconds. Dip each tortilla in the sauce to coat it lightly, then spoon about ¼ cup of the tempeh mixture in a line down the center. Roll the tortilla up around the filling. Set the filled tortilla in the prepared baking dish, seam-side down. Repeat with the remaining tortillas and filling.
4. Spoon the remaining sauce over the top, covering all of the tortillas. Sprinkle the cheese over the top, if using, and bake in the preheated oven for about 40 minutes, until heated through and bubbling. Serve immediately.

Nutrition Info:
- Calories: 724; Protein: 38g; Total Fat: 35g; Saturated Fat: 12g; Carbohydrates: 76g; Fiber: 15g; Sodium: 998mg;

Eggplant And Chickpea Curry

Servings: 4 | Cooking Time: 15 Minutes

Ingredients:
- 2 tablespoons Garlic Oil
- 6 scallions, green parts only, minced
- 2 cups chopped eggplant
- 1 cup canned chickpeas, drained
- 1 cup unsweetened almond milk
- 1 tablespoon curry powder
- ¼ teaspoon freshly ground black pepper

Directions:
1. In a large skillet over medium-high heat, heat the garlic oil until it shimmers.
2. Add the scallions and eggplant. Cook for about 5 minutes, stirring, until the eggplant is soft.
3. Add the chickpeas, almond milk, curry powder, and pepper. Bring to a boil. Reduce the heat to medium-low and simmer for 10 minutes.

Nutrition Info:
- Calories: 275; Total Fat: 11g; Saturated Fat: 1g; Carbohydrates: 36g; Fiber: 12g; Sodium: 62mg; Protein: 11g

Zucchini Pasta Alla Puttanesca

Servings:4 | Cooking Time: 15 Minutes

Ingredients:
- 2 tablespoons olive oil
- 1½ cups diced tomatoes
- 1 tablespoon Garlic Oil (here)
- 2 tablespoons chopped Kalamata olives
- 1 tablespoon capers, drained
- 1 teaspoon salt
- ½ teaspoon freshly ground black pepper
- ½ teaspoon red pepper flakes
- ¼ cup chopped fresh basil
- 3 large zucchini, cut into ribbons with a spiral slicer
- ½ cup freshly grated Parmesan cheese

Directions:
1. Heat the olive oil in a large skillet over medium-high heat. Add the tomatoes and Garlic Oil, and cook for about 10 minutes, until the tomatoes begin to break down and become saucy. Add the olives, capers, salt, pepper, and red pepper flakes, and cook for 5 minutes more. Stir in the basil.
2. Remove the pan from the heat and add the zucchini. Toss until the zucchini noodles soften and are well coated with the sauce. Serve immediately, garnished with Parmesan cheese.

Nutrition Info:
- Calories: 226; Protein: 14g; Total Fat: 15g; Saturated Fat: 5g; Carbohydrates: 16g; Fiber: 5g; Sodium: 974mg;

Lemon And Mozzarella Polenta Pizza

Servings:4 | Cooking Time:x

Ingredients:
- For the crust:
- 1 tablespoon extra-virgin olive oil
- 2 1/2 cups vegetable stock (or use water)
- 1 1/4 teaspoons salt, divided
- 1 cup coarse cornmeal
- 1 tablespoon garlic-infused olive oil
- 2 teaspoons freshly ground black pepper
- For the pizza topping:
- 1/2 pound mozzarella, cut into small cubes
- 1 small lemon, cut into thin slices
- 5 large leaves fresh basil, chopped
- 1 teaspoon truffle salt
- 1 teaspoon freshly ground black pepper

Directions:
1. Preheat oven to 450ºF. Brush olive oil on a pizza pan or baking sheet.
2. In a medium saucepan over medium-high heat, add stock or water and 1/4 teaspoon salt. Bring just about to a boil, reduce heat to medium, and add cornmeal. Turn heat to low and simmer, whisking frequently for about 10–15 minutes. Polenta needs to be thick, so add more water only if needed.
3. Stir garlic-infused oil into polenta. Quickly spread polenta out onto prepared pan, into a thickness of about 1/2". Sprinkle with 1 teaspoon salt and pepper. Cover baking sheet with plastic wrap and place in refrigerator until firm, about 1 hour. Can be refrigerated overnight.
4. Place polenta in oven and bake 25–30 minutes or until brown and crisp on edges.
5. Take polenta out of oven, sprinkle with mozzarella cheese, then spread lemon and basil on top. Sprinkle with truffle salt and pepper. Put pizza back in oven 2–4 minutes or until cheese has melted. Cut into square or triangle slices and serve hot or at room temperature.

Nutrition Info:
- Calories: 364,Fat: 20g,Protein: 15g,Sodium: 1,685mg,-Carbohydrates: 31.

Summer Vegetable Pasta

Servings:4 | Cooking Time:x

Ingredients:
- 1 pound gluten-free penne pasta, cooked and drained
- 2 1/2 tablespoons extra-virgin olive oil, divided
- 1 medium eggplant, diced into 1/2" cubes
- 1 medium zucchini, sliced lengthwise into 1/4"-thick planks
- 1 cup halved grape tomatoes
- 1 tablespoon garlic-infused olive oil
- 2 tablespoons lemon juice
- 1 tablespoon rice wine vinegar
- 1 teaspoon fresh dill
- 1 medium cucumber, peeled and cut into quarters
- 2 tablespoons chopped fresh basil leaves
- 1 tablespoon chopped fresh cilantro leaves
- 1 teaspoon salt
- 1 teaspoon freshly ground black pepper

Directions:
1. Place penne in a large salad bowl and add 1/2 tablespoon extra-virgin olive oil. Toss noodles gently to coat.
2. Heat a wok or large frying pan to medium heat. Add eggplant, zucchini, and tomatoes. Sauté until slightly tender. Transfer to salad bowl with pasta.
3. Make the dressing: Combine remaining olive oil, garlic-infused oil, lemon juice, vinegar, and dill in a food processor and blend until smooth. Set aside.
4. Toss cucumber, basil, cilantro, salt, and black pepper into salad bowl. Add dressing. Toss until all ingredients are evenly distributed.

Nutrition Info:
- Calories: 577,Fat: 14g,Protein: 17g,Sodium: 608mg,Carbohydrates: 97.

Vegetable And Rice Noodle Bowl

Servings:2 | Cooking Time:x

Ingredients:
- For the teriyaki sauce:
- 1/4 cup rice wine vinegar
- 1 tablespoon sesame oil
- 1 tablespoon light brown sugar
- 1/16 teaspoon wheat-free asafetida powder
- 1 1/2 teaspoons minced fresh gingerroot
- 1/4 teaspoon red pepper flakes
- 1 teaspoon freshly ground black pepper
- For the noodles:
- 1 tablespoon coconut oil
- 2 cups finely chopped broccoli florets
- 1 small stalk celery, chopped
- 2 medium carrots, peeled and shredded
- 3 ounces rice noodles, cooked and drained
- 1 scallion, chopped, green part only
- 2 teaspoons toasted sesame seeds

Directions:
1. In a medium bowl, whisk together all sauce ingredients until combined. Set aside.
2. Preheat a wok over medium-high heat. Add oil to coat pan. Add broccoli, celery, carrots, and 2 tablespoons of teriyaki sauce. Sauté about 8 minutes.
3. Stir drained noodles into wok along with remaining teriyaki sauce. Cook 2–3 minutes and serve immediately garnished with scallions and sesame seeds.

Nutrition Info:
- Calories: 281,Fat: 16g,Protein: 4g,Sodium: 92mg,Carbohydrates: 32.

Baked Tofu Báhn Mì Lettuce Wrap

Servings:4 | Cooking Time: 20 Minutes

Ingredients:
- FOR THE TOFU
- 1 (16-ounce) package firm tofu, drained and cut into ½-inch-thick slabs
- 2 tablespoons gluten-free soy sauce
- 2 teaspoons grated fresh ginger
- Vegetable oil or coconut oil to prepare the baking sheet
- FOR THE VEGETABLES
- ½ cup rice vinegar
- ¼ cup water
- ¼ cup sugar
- 1 teaspoon salt
- 1½ cups shredded carrot
- 1½ cups shredded daikon radish
- FOR THE WRAPS
- 8 large lettuce leaves
- 2 tablespoons mayonnaise
- ½ medium cucumber, peeled, seeded, and cut into matchsticks
- 2 large jalapeño chiles, thinly sliced
- 1 cup cilantro leaves

Directions:
1. Line a rimmed baking sheet with paper towels and place the cut tofu on the sheet in a single layer. Top with another layer of paper towels and then another baking sheet. Weight the top baking sheet down with something heavy (cans of tomatoes or beans work well). Let sit for 30 minutes.
2. While the tofu is draining, prepare the vegetables. In a small saucepan, combine the vinegar, water, sugar, and salt and cook, stirring, over medium heat, until the sugar has dissolved, for about 3 minutes. Remove the pan from the heat and add the carrot and daikon, stirring to coat well. Let sit for 20 minutes.
3. In a large bowl, combine the soy sauce and ginger. Add the pressed tofu and toss to coat well.
4. Let the tofu sit for about 15 minutes, and preheat the oven to 350°F.
5. Oil a large baking sheet with vegetable or coconut oil.
6. Arrange the tofu slabs in a single layer on the prepared baking sheet and bake in the preheated oven for about 10 minutes. Turn the pieces over and bake for another 10 minutes, until the tofu is browned. Remove from the oven and cut into 1-inch-wide sticks.
7. To make the wraps, arrange the lettuce leaves on your work surface and spread a bit of mayonnaise on each, dividing equally. Fill with the baked tofu, cucumber, chiles, and cilantro. Drain the pickled carrots and daikon, and place a handful onto each wrap. Serve immediately.

Nutrition Info:
- Calories: 180; Protein: 6g; Total Fat: 3g; Saturated Fat: 0g; Carbohydrates: 28g; Fiber: 2g; Sodium: 4138mg;

Pasta With Pesto Sauce

Servings:4 | Cooking Time: 0 Minutes

Ingredients:
- 8 ounces gluten-free angel hair pasta, cooked according to the package instructions. Drained
- 1 recipe Macadamia Spinach Pesto
- ¼ cup grated Parmesan cheese

Directions:
1. In the warm pot that you used to cook the pasta, toss the noodles with the pesto.
2. Sprinkle with the cheese.

Nutrition Info:
- Calories:449; Total Fat: 25g; Saturated Fat: 6g; Carbohydrates: 46g; Fiber: 3g; Sodium: 444mg; Protein: 13g

Tempeh Lettuce Wraps

Servings:4 | Cooking Time: 8 Minutes

Ingredients:
- 2 tablespoons Garlic Oil
- 4 cups chopped tempeh
- 1 tablespoon Chinese five-spice powder
- ¼ cup creamy sugar-free natural peanut butter
- ¼ cup Low-FODMAP Vegetable Broth
- 1 tablespoon gluten-free soy sauce
- 1 teaspoon ground ginger
- 8 large lettuce leaves
- Minced scallions, green parts only, for garnishing (optional)
- Chopped fresh cilantro leaves, for garnishing (optional)
- Bean sprouts, for garnishing (optional)
- Chopped peanuts, for garnishing (optional)

Directions:
1. In a large skillet over medium-high heat, heat the garlic oil until it shimmers.
2. Add the tempeh and five-spice powder. Cook for 3 to 4 minutes, stirring, until the tempeh is warmed through.
3. In a small bowl, whisk the peanut butter, broth, soy sauce, and ginger. Stir the sauce into the tempeh. Cook for 3 minutes more, stirring.
4. Serve with the lettuce leaves to wrap and the garnishes (if using) on the side.

Nutrition Info:
- Calories:433; Total Fat: 27g; Saturated Fat: 6g; Carbohydrates: 21g; Fiber: 2g; Sodium: 367mg; Protein: 36g

Mediterranean Noodles

Servings:4 | Cooking Time:x

Ingredients:
- 1 medium eggplant
- ½ cup garlic-infused olive oil
- ½ teaspoon sea salt
- 2 teaspoons freshly ground black pepper
- 1 (12-ounce) package gluten-free fusilli, cooked, drained, and rinsed under cold water
- 20 grape tomatoes, halved
- ½ cup sliced black olives
- 20 fresh basil leaves, torn
- 1 teaspoon dried oregano
- Juice of 2 medium lemons
- ½ cup grated Parmesan cheese

Directions:
1. Preheat oven to 475°F.
2. Cut eggplant into chunks and place in a large bowl. Using your hands, toss eggplant with oil, salt, and black pepper.
3. Place eggplant in a single layer on a baking sheet. Bake 20 minutes, flipping halfway through baking. When done, remove from oven and allow to cool. Eggplant should be soft. Transfer back to large bowl along with cooked noodles.
4. Stir in tomatoes, olives, basil, oregano, lemon juice, and Parmesan and serve.

Nutrition Info:
- Calories: 470,Fat: 33g,Protein: 11g,Sodium: 680mg,Carbohydrates: 36.

Mixed Grains, Seeds, And Vegetable Bowl

Servings:4 | Cooking Time:x

Ingredients:
- 2 medium sweet potatoes, peeled and cut into 2" chunks
- 2 tablespoons olive oil
- 1½ tablespoons balsamic vinegar
- ½ teaspoon dried rosemary
- ½ teaspoon dried thyme
- ½ teaspoon dried oregano
- 2 tablespoons pumpkin seeds
- 1⅓ of a whole fennel bulb, halved lengthwise and cut into quarters
- ½ cup brown rice, cooked
- ¾ cup red quinoa, rinsed and cooked
- 1 cup buckwheat, rinsed and cooked
- ½ tablespoon coconut oil
- 3 cups baby spinach

Directions:
1. Preheat oven to 375°F.
2. Place sweet potatoes in a medium bowl. Add oil, vinegar, rosemary, thyme, and oregano. Toss with hands to coat. Place on rimmed baking sheet and roast 1 hour, flipping halfway through cooking and adding pumpkin seeds and fennel.
3. Add rice, quinoa, and buckwheat to same bowl used to prepare sweet potatoes. Stir in coconut oil.
4. Once sweet potatoes have finished baking and are tender, immediately add to bowl. Add spinach and toss. Serve immediately.

Nutrition Info:
- Calories: 411,Fat: 14g,Protein: 12g,Sodium: 72mg,Carbohydrates: 63.

Turmeric Rice With Cranberries

Servings:2 | Cooking Time:x

Ingredients:
- ½ cup no-sugar-added dried cranberries
- 2 cups lukewarm water
- 1 tablespoon coconut oil
- 2 tablespoons pine nuts
- ½ teaspoon ground turmeric
- 1/16 teaspoon wheat-free asafetida powder
- ½ teaspoon saffron dissolved in ¼ cup hot water
- 2 tablespoons light brown sugar
- ¼ teaspoon sea salt
- 1 cup cooked basmati rice

Directions:
1. Soak cranberries in lukewarm water for about 10 minutes to plump. Drain.
2. In a wok or medium skillet on medium-high, heat coconut oil and stir in cranberries and pine nuts. Add turmeric, asafetida, saffron, sugar, and salt and reduce heat to low; cook 7 minutes.
3. Add rice and stir until evenly coated; serve immediately.

Nutrition Info:
- Calories: 396,Fat: 16g,Protein: 4g,Sodium: 307mg,Carbohydrates: 63.

Vegan Potato Salad, Cypriot-style
Servings:6 | Cooking Time:x

Ingredients:
- 2 1/2 pounds Cyprus or Yukon Gold potatoes, peeled
- Juice of 1 medium lemon
- 2 tablespoons extra-virgin olive oil
- 1/2 teaspoon sea salt
- 1 teaspoon freshly ground black pepper
- 1 tablespoon dried oregano
- 1 bunch fresh cilantro, roughly chopped
- 1/4 cup chopped fresh flat-leaf parsley
- 3 scallions, chopped, green part only
- 1 tablespoon olive oil
- 1/4 cup roughly chopped black olives
- 2 tablespoons capers, rinsed and drained

Directions:
1. In a shallow pan of salted boiling water, cook potatoes 25 minutes. Drain and set aside until cool, then slice into small chunks.
2. Place potatoes in a large bowl with lemon juice and extra-virgin olive oil. Add salt, pepper, and oregano. Toss to coat evenly.
3. Add cilantro, parsley, and scallions. Toss to mix.
4. Heat olive oil in a small skillet over medium heat. Add olives and capers and fry 3 minutes. Sprinkle over potatoes in bowl. Tastes best when served immediately, but can be stored in refrigerator in an airtight container up to 2 days.

Nutrition Info:
- Calories: 203,Fat: 8g,Protein: 4g,Sodium: 345mg,Carbohydrates: 32.

Baked Tofu And Vegetables
Servings:4 | Cooking Time:x

Ingredients:
- 2 (14-ounce) packages extra-firm tofu, pressed between paper towels and patted dry
- 2 tablespoons toasted sesame oil, divided
- 2 teaspoons sesame seeds
- 2 1/2 tablespoons gluten-free soy sauce (tamari), divided
- 7–8 cups chopped bok choy (about 8 stalks)
- 1 bunch scallions, diced, green part only
- 1 medium red bell pepper, seeded and diced
- 1/4 cup slivered almonds
- 2 tablespoons rice wine vinegar

Directions:
1. Preheat oven to 400°F. Grease a large rimmed baking sheet with cooking spray.
2. Cut tofu into 1" pieces and toss in a large bowl with 1 tablespoon sesame oil, sesame seeds, and 2 tablespoons soy sauce.
3. Spread in a single layer on the prepared baking sheet. Bake tofu on lower rack of oven. Bake until browned, 25–30 minutes, flipping once.
4. While tofu is baking, heat a large skillet on medium-high and coat with 1 tablespoon sesame oil.
5. Add bok choy, scallions, bell pepper, almonds, remaining 1/2 tablespoon soy sauce, and vinegar. Cook until bok choy is slightly tender, stirring frequently. Place in same bowl used to prepare tofu.
6. Once tofu is ready, add to vegetables in bowl and stir until combined. Divide into 4 bowls and serve.

Nutrition Info:
- Calories: 267,Fat: 16g,Protein: 18g,Sodium: 725mg,Carbohydrates: 12.

Vegetable Fried Rice
Servings:2 | Cooking Time:x

Ingredients:
- 2 large eggs
- 1 tablespoon sesame oil
- 1/2 medium carrot, peeled and thinly sliced
- 1/2 medium red bell pepper, seeded and diced
- 1 teaspoon palm sugar
- 1/16 teaspoon wheat-free asafetida powder
- 1 tablespoon gluten-free soy sauce (tamari)
- 1 teaspoon gluten-free fish sauce
- 1 tablespoon rice wine vinegar
- 1 large green onion, chopped, green part only
- 1 tablespoon freshly grated gingerroot
- 1 cup cooked brown rice
- 2 cups baby spinach

Directions:
1. Whisk eggs in a small bowl. Heat a wok or medium skillet on medium-high; spray with cooking spray and add eggs to pan. Cook 4–5 minutes or until eggs are cooked but still slightly moist. Set eggs aside on cutting board.
2. Add sesame oil to pan, then add carrot and bell pepper. Cook about 3 minutes, stirring occasionally.
3. Meanwhile, in a small bowl, stir together sugar, asafetida, soy sauce, fish sauce, and vinegar until sugar is dissolved.
4. Add green onion to pan and stir 1 minute; add ginger and cook 1 more minute.
5. Add rice and cook 2 minutes, stirring. Add soy sauce mixture and continue stirring until absorbed into rice, about 2 minutes.

6. Add spinach and cook until wilted, about 3 minutes. Coarsely chop egg and stir into rice.

Nutrition Info:
- Calories: 296,Fat: 13g,Protein: 11g,Sodium: 790mg,Carbohydrates: 35.

Watercress Zucchini Soup

Servings:4 | Cooking Time: 15 Minutes

Ingredients:
- 2 tablespoons extra-virgin olive oil
- 1 leek, white part removed and the greens finely chopped
- 3 cups homemade (onion- and garlic-free) vegetable broth
- 1 pound zucchini, chopped
- 8 ounces chopped watercress
- 2 tablespoons dried tarragon
- 1 teaspoon salt
- ¼ teaspoon freshly ground black pepper
- 2 tablespoons heavy cream

Directions:
1. In a large pot, heat the olive oil over medium-high heat until it shimmers.
2. Add the leek greens and cook, stirring occasionally, until the vegetables are soft, about seven minutes.
3. Add the vegetable broth and zucchini and simmer, stirring occasionally, for eight minutes.
4. Add the watercress, tarragon, salt, and pepper. Cook, stirring occasionally, an additional five minutes.
5. Carefully transfer the soup mixture to a blender or food processor. You may need to work in batches.
6. Fold a towel and place it over the top of the blender with your hand on top of it. Purée the soup for 30 seconds, and then remove the lid to vent steam. Close the blender and purée for another 30 seconds, until the mixture is smooth.
7. Transfer the mixture back to the cooking pot and stir in the heavy cream. Serve immediately.

Nutrition Info:
- Calories: 161; Total Fat: 11g; Saturated Fat: 3g; Cholesterol: 10mg; Carbohydrates: 9g; Fiber: 2g; Protein: 7g;

Latin Quinoa-stuffed Peppers

Servings:4 | Cooking Time:x

Ingredients:
- 1/2 cup quinoa
- 1 cup Vegetable Stock (see Chapter 4)
- 3 tablespoons nutritional yeast
- 2 cups spinach
- 2 teaspoons ground cumin
- 1 tablespoon chili powder
- 1 cup whole-kernel corn, drained
- 2 tablespoons macadamia nuts
- 4 large red, yellow, green, or orange bell peppers, tops cut off, seeds removed, halved
- 2 tablespoons coconut oil
- 1/2 ripe medium avocado, sliced into eighths
- 1 tablespoon fresh lime juice

Directions:
1. Preheat oven to 375°F and lightly grease a 9" × 13" baking dish or rimmed baking sheet with cooking spray.
2. Combine quinoa with stock in a medium saucepan. Bring to a boil. Cover, reduce heat to low, and simmer 15 minutes or until quinoa is tender.
3. Add cooked quinoa to a large mixing bowl and thoroughly mix together with yeast, spinach, cumin, chili powder, corn, and macadamia nuts.
4. Place peppers in baking dish and brush with coconut oil. Stuff peppers with quinoa mixture. Make sure none of the spinach is showing. Cover dish with foil.
5. Bake 30 minutes, then remove foil and increase heat to 400°F; bake another 30 minutes.
6. Top with avocado, then lime juice. Serve immediately.

Nutrition Info:
- Calories: 418,Fat: 22g,Protein: 14g,Sodium: 1,188mg,Carbohydrates: 46.

Tofu Burger Patties

Servings:4 | Cooking Time: 10 Minutes

Ingredients:
- 8 ounces firm tofu, mashed with a fork
- 4 scallions, green parts only, minced
- 1 cup rolled oats
- 1 egg, beaten
- 2 teaspoons ground cumin
- 2 teaspoons chili powder
- ½ teaspoon sea salt
- ¼ teaspoon freshly ground black pepper
- Nonstick cooking spray

Directions:
1. In a medium bowl, stir together the tofu, scallions, oats, egg, cumin, chili powder, salt, and pepper. Form the mixture into 4 patties.
2. Spray a large nonstick skillet with cooking spray and place it over medium-high heat.
3. Add the patties and cook for about 5 minutes per side, until browned on both sides.

Nutrition Info:
- Calories:146; Total Fat: 5g; Saturated Fat: 1g; Carbohydrates: 17g; Fiber: 4g; Sodium: 275mg; Protein: 10g

Moroccan-spiced Lentil And Quinoa Stew

Servings: 4 | Cooking Time: 30 Minutes

Ingredients:
- 1 tablespoon olive oil
- 4 carrots, diced
- 1 leek (green part only), halved lengthwise and thinly sliced
- 1 tablespoon Garlic Oil (here)
- 1 teaspoon ground cumin
- 1 teaspoon ground coriander
- 1 teaspoon ground turmeric
- ¼ teaspoon ground cinnamon
- 1½ teaspoons salt
- ¼ teaspoon freshly ground black pepper
- 8 cups homemade (onion- and garlic-free) vegetable broth
- ¾ cup uncooked quinoa, rinsed
- 1¾ cups canned lentils
- 1 (28-ounce) can onion- and garlic-free diced tomatoes, drained
- 2 tablespoons tomato paste
- 4 cups chopped fresh spinach or 1 (10-ounce) package frozen chopped spinach, thawed
- ½ cup chopped fresh cilantro
- 2 tablespoons lemon juice

Directions:
1. Heat the olive oil in a medium stockpot set over medium heat. Add the carrots and leek, and cook, stirring frequently, for about 10 minutes, until the carrots soften. Add the Garlic Oil, cumin, coriander, turmeric, cinnamon, salt, and pepper. Cook, stirring, for about 1 minute more.
2. Stir in the broth, quinoa, lentils, tomatoes, and tomato paste, and bring the mixture to a boil. Reduce the heat to low and simmer, stirring occasionally, for about 20 minutes, until the quinoa is tender.
3. Stir in the spinach and cook for 5 minutes more.
4. Stir in the cilantro and lemon juice, and serve immediately.

Nutrition Info:
- Calories: 638; Protein: 43g; Total Fat: 11g; Saturated Fat: 2g; Carbohydrates: 97g; Fiber: 36g; Sodium: 2541mg;

Chipotle Tofu And Sweet Potato Tacos With Avocado Salsa

Servings: 4 | Cooking Time: 20 Minutes

Ingredients:
- FOR THE FILLING
- 2 tablespoons olive oil
- 2 sweet potatoes, peeled and cut into ½-inch cubes
- 1 pound firm tofu, diced
- ½ to 1 teaspoon ground chipotle chiles
- 2 tablespoons sugar
- Juice of 1 lime
- FOR THE AVOCADO SALSA
- 2 tomatoes
- ½ avocado, diced
- ¼ serrano chile, diced
- Juice of ½ lime
- ¼ teaspoon salt
- 2 tablespoons chopped fresh cilantro
- TO SERVE
- 8 soft corn tortillas

Directions:
1. Heat the olive oil in a large skillet over medium heat. Add the sweet potatoes and cook for about 5 minutes, until the potatoes begin to soften. Add the tofu, chipotle, sugar, and lime juice. Reduce the heat to low and cook, stirring occasionally, until the sweet potatoes are tender, about 15 minutes.
2. Meanwhile, wrap the tortillas in aluminum foil and heat them in a 350°F oven for 10 minutes.
3. To make the avocado salsa, combine the tomatoes, avocado, chile, lime juice, and salt in a medium bowl. Stir in the cilantro.
4. To serve, fill the tortillas with the filliing, dividing equally, and spoon a dollop of avocado salsa on top of each. Serve immediately.

Nutrition Info:
- Calories: 421; Protein: 15g; Total Fat: 18g; Saturated Fat: 3g; Carbohydrates: 55g; Fiber: 10g; Sodium: 229mg;

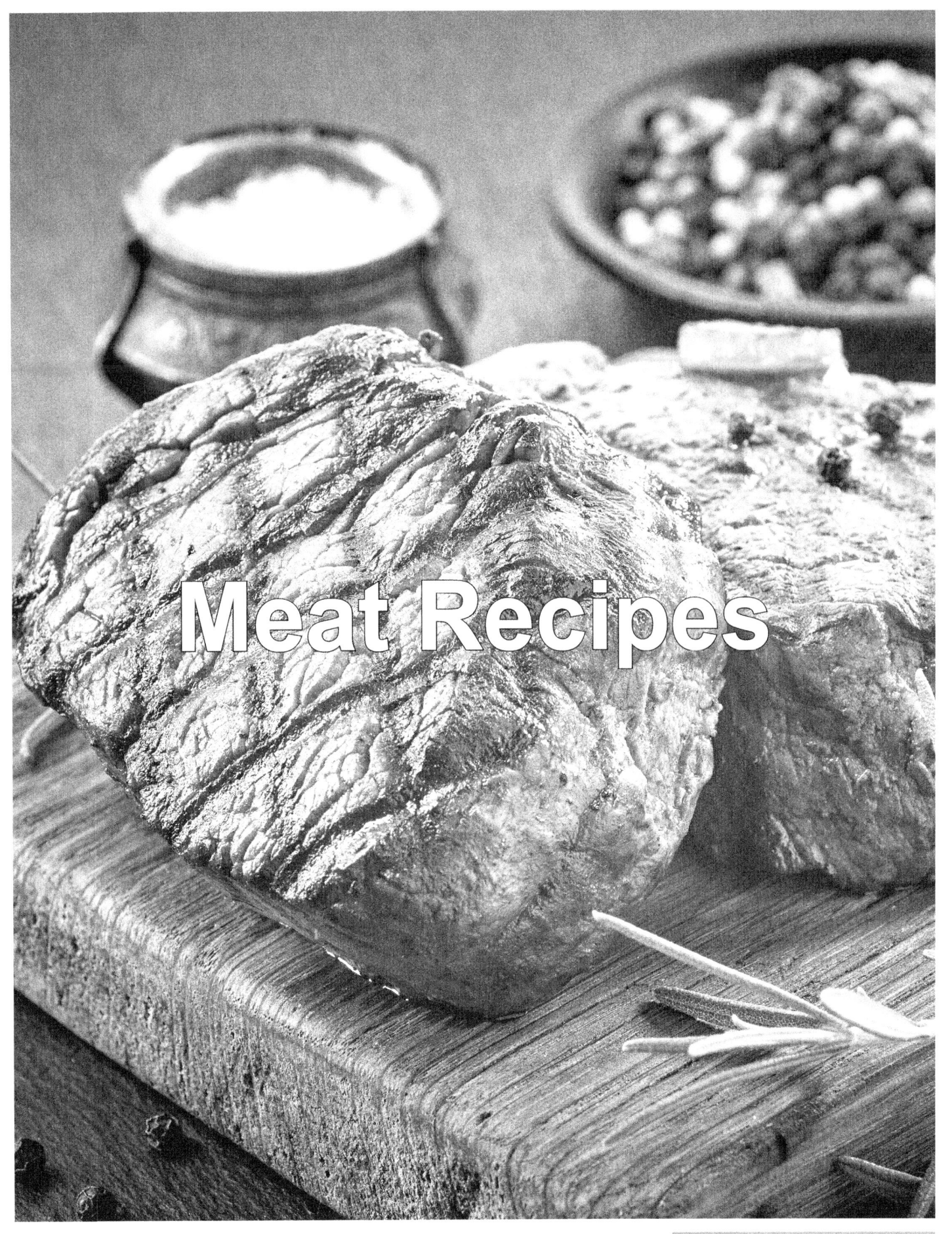

Meat Recipes

Meat Recipes

Grilled Chicken Parmigiana

Servings:4 | Cooking Time:x

Ingredients:
- 1 pound skinless, boneless chicken breast, cut into thin cutlets
- 1/2 cup Traditional Tomato Sauce (see recipe in Chapter 9)
- 16 fresh basil leaves, sliced into thin strips
- 8 ounces mozzarella cheese, thinly sliced

Directions:
1. Heat a charcoal or gas grill to 350°F. Cook chicken 3 minutes per side or until cooked through.
2. With chicken still on grill, place 1 tablespoon of sauce and a small pile of basil on top of each cutlet. Cover with 2 mozzarella slices. Continue to grill until cheese has melted, approximately 3 minutes. Serve.

Nutrition Info:
- Calories: 303,Fat: 15g,Protein: 37g,Sodium: 642mg,Carbohydrates: 3.

Mild Lamb Curry

Servings:6 | Cooking Time:x

Ingredients:
- ½ cup (75 g) cornstarch
- 2 pounds 10 ounces (1.2 kg) lean lamb steaks, cut into ¾-inch (2 cm) pieces
- 2 teaspoons garlic-infused olive oil
- 2 tablespoons rice bran oil or sunflower oil
- 2 teaspoons ground cinnamon
- 2 heaping tablespoons ground cumin
- 2 teaspoons ground ginger
- 1 heaping tablespoon ground turmeric
- 2 teaspoons paprika
- 1 teaspoon cayenne pepper
- 1 teaspoon salt
- 1 teaspoon freshly ground black pepper
- 4 cups (1 liter) gluten-free, onion-free beef stock*
- 2 heaping tablespoons light brown sugar
- One 14.5-ounce (425 g) can crushed tomatoes
- Steamed rice and cilantro leaves, for serving

Directions:
1. Place the cornstarch in a shallow bowl. Add the lamb pieces and toss to coat well. Shake off any excess.
2. Heat the garlic-infused oil and rice bran oil in a large heavy-bottomed saucepan or Dutch oven over medium heat. Add the cinnamon, cumin, ginger, turmeric, paprika, cayenne, salt, and pepper and cook for 1 to 2 minutes, until fragrant. Add the lamb and cook, stirring occasionally, for 5 to 7 minutes, until nicely browned. Add the stock and brown sugar and bring to a boil, then reduce the heat and simmer gently for 1½ hours, stirring occasionally.
3. Stir in the crushed tomatoes and cook for another hour or until the meat is very tender. Make sure the heat is kept very low so the lamb does not boil dry. (Add a little water if necessary.)
4. Season to taste with salt and pepper and serve with steamed rice, garnished with cilantro.

Nutrition Info:
- 538 calories; 27 g protein; 39 g total fat; 15 g saturated fat; 16 g carbohydrates; 2 g fiber; 647 mg sodium

Chili-rubbed Pork Chops With Raspberry Sauce

Servings:4 | Cooking Time: 10 Minutes

Ingredients:
- 2 teaspoons gluten-free, onion- and garlic-free chili powder
- ½ teaspoon salt
- 1 teaspoon chopped fresh thyme
- 4 (6-ounce) bone-in, center-cut pork chops (about ½-inch thick)
- 2 tablespoons olive oil
- ¼ cup homemade (onion- and garlic-free) chicken broth
- 2 tablespoons seedless raspberry preserves

Directions:
1. In a small bowl, combine the chili powder, salt, and thyme. Coat the pork chops all over with the spice mixture.
2. Heat the oil in a large skillet over medium-high heat. Cook the chops for about 3 minutes per side, until they are browned and cooked through. Transfer the cooked chops to a large plate or serving platter, tent loosely with foil, and keep warm.
3. Add the broth to the skillet and cook, stirring and scraping up any browned bits from the bottom of the pan, for about 30 seconds. Add the preserves and cook, stirring constantly, for 1 minute or until the sauce thickens.
4. Serve the pork chops brushed with the glaze.

Nutrition Info:
- Calories: 286; Protein: 35g; Total Fat: 14g; Saturated Fat: 3g; Carbohydrates: 7g; Fiber: 0g; Sodium: 657mg;

Chinese Chicken

Servings: 4 | Cooking Time: x

Ingredients:
- ¾ cup arrowroot powder
- 1/2 cup white wine, divided
- 1/2 cup gluten-free tamari, divided
- 1 pound boneless, skinless chicken breasts, cubed
- 1/2 teaspoon sugar
- 1/2 cup Basic Roast Chicken Stock (see recipe in Chapter 8)
- 2 tablespoons sesame oil, divided
- 1 teaspoon natural peanut butter
- 4 garlic cloves, peeled and slightly smashed
- 1 cup broccoli florets
- 1 cup sliced red bell pepper
- 2 cups cooked brown rice

Directions:
1. In a medium bowl, stir to combine arrowroot and 1/4 cup each of wine and tamari. Add chicken; stir to coat. Cover and refrigerate for 30 minutes.
2. Transfer chicken to a colander and drain marinade completely. Set chicken aside.
3. In a separate bowl, combine sugar, stock, and remaining wine and tamari.
4. In another small bowl, whisk 1 tablespoon oil and peanut butter.
5. Heat remaining oil over medium-high heat in a large wok or skillet. Add the garlic and sauté, stirring constantly, until softened and brown at the edges, about 2 minutes. Remove garlic from pan and discard, leaving oil.
6. Add chicken and stir-fry quickly, browning chicken on all sides—approximately 8–10 minutes. (Lower heat if chicken is browning too quickly.) Scrape up and discard any loose marinade bits. Once fully cooked through, transfer chicken to a plate and cover to keep warm.
7. Add broccoli and bell pepper to skillet and quickly stir-fry for 1 minute. Add stock and peanut butter mixtures and stir. Cover, then lower heat and simmer for 5–8 minutes, until vegetables are crisp-tender.
8. Divide rice, chicken, and vegetables in their sauce evenly among four plates and serve.

Nutrition Info:
- Calories: 458, Fat: 11g, Protein: 30g, Sodium: 2,014mg, Carbohydrates: 53.

Orange-ginger Salmon

Servings: 4 | Cooking Time: 12 Minutes

Ingredients:
- ¼ cup Garlic Oil
- Juice of 2 oranges
- 2 tablespoons gluten-free soy sauce
- 1 tablespoon peeled and grated fresh ginger
- 1 pound salmon fillet, quartered

Directions:
1. Preheat the oven to 450°F.
2. In a shallow baking dish, whisk together the garlic oil, orange juice, soy sauce, and ginger.
3. Place the salmon, flesh-side down, in the marinade. Marinate for 10 minutes.
4. Place the salmon, skin-side up, on a rimmed baking sheet. Bake for 12 to 15 minutes, until opaque.

Nutrition Info:
- Calories: 282; Total Fat: 20g; Saturated Fat: 3g; Carbohydrates: 5g; Fiber: 0g; Sodium: 553mg; Protein: 23g

Creamy Smoked Salmon Pasta

Servings: 4 | Cooking Time: 9 Minutes

Ingredients:
- 2 tablespoons Garlic Oil
- 6 scallions, green parts only, chopped
- 2 tablespoons capers, drained
- 12 ounces smoked salmon, flaked
- ¾ cup unsweetened almond milk
- 2 tablespoons chopped fresh dill
- ⅛ teaspoon freshly ground black pepper
- 8 ounces gluten-free pasta, cooked according to the package directions and drained

Directions:
1. In a large nonstick skillet over medium-high heat, heat the garlic oil until it shimmers.
2. Add the scallions and capers. Cook for 2 minutes, stirring.
3. Add the salmon and cook for 2 minutes more.
4. Stir in the almond milk, dill, and pepper. Simmer for 3 minutes.
5. Toss with the hot pasta.

Nutrition Info:
- Calories: 287; Total Fat: 6g; Saturated Fat: 1g; Carbohydrates: 35g; Fiber: 1g; Sodium: 1,920mg; Protein: 23g

Spicy Pulled Pork

Servings:8 | Cooking Time: 6 Hours

Ingredients:
- FOR THE PORK
- 3 tablespoons paprika
- 1 tablespoon brown sugar
- 1 tablespoon dry mustard
- 3 tablespoons salt
- 1 pork shoulder or butt roast (about 5 pounds)
- FOR THE SAUCE
- 1½ cups white-wine vinegar
- 1 cup onion- and garlic-free mustard
- ⅓ cup onion- and garlic-free tomato sauce
- ½ cup packed brown sugar
- 1 tablespoon Garlic Oil (here)
- 1 teaspoon salt
- 1 teaspoon cayenne
- ½ teaspoon freshly ground black pepper

Directions:
1. To prepare the roast, in a small bowl, combine the paprika, brown sugar, dry mustard, and salt.
2. Rub the spice blend all over the pork. Cover and refrigerate for at least 1 hour or as long as overnight.
3. Preheat the oven to 300°F.
4. Roast the pork in a roasting pan in the preheated oven for 6 hours, until the meat is falling apart (a meat thermometer should read about 170°F).
5. While the pork is in the oven, prepare the sauce. In a medium saucepan, combine the vinegar, mustard, tomato sauce, brown sugar, Garlic Oil, salt, cayenne, and black pepper, and bring to a simmer over medium heat. Cook, stirring occasionally, until the sugar is completely dissolved, for about 10 minutes. Remove from the heat.
6. When the pork is done, remove it from the oven and let it rest for about 10 minutes. While the pork is still warm, shred the meat using two forks. Place the shredded meat in a large bowl and mix in half of the sauce.
7. Serve warm, topped with additional sauce.

Nutrition Info:
- Calories: 988; Protein: 72g; Total Fat: 67g; Saturated Fat: 23g; Carbohydrates: 20g; Fiber: 4g; Sodium: 3167mg;

Baked Chicken And Mozzarella Croquettes

Servings:4 | Cooking Time:x

Ingredients:
- Nonstick cooking spray
- 5 large boneless, skinless chicken thighs, excess fat removed, cut into chunks
- ⅔ cup (80 g) dried gluten-free, soy-free bread crumbs*
- 1 large egg
- ¼ cup (60 ml) Basil Pesto
- 4 ounces (115 g) mozzarella, cut into 8 cubes
- 8 basil leaves
- 8 prosciutto slices (optional)
- ¼ cup (60 ml) light cream
- 1 teaspoon garlic-infused olive oil
- Salt and freshly ground black pepper
- Green salad or vegetables, for serving

Directions:
1. Preheat the oven to 350°F (180°C). Grease a baking sheet with nonstick cooking spray.
2. Combine the chicken, bread crumbs, egg, and pesto in a food processor or blender and process until just combined—do not puree. Divide the mixture into 8 portions and form into balls. Gently flatten each ball and place a piece of mozzarella and a basil leaf in the middle of each. Re-form the balls to enclose the cheese and basil, then shape into croquettes about 2 inches (5 cm) long and 1 inch (3 cm) wide. If using the prosciutto, wrap each croquette in a slice and secure with a toothpick.
3. Place the croquettes on the baking sheet. Bake for 20 minutes, or until the chicken is cooked through (and the prosciutto, if using, is crisp). Test by cutting into a croquette; it should be opaque.
4. Meanwhile, to make the sauce, combine the cream and garlic-infused oil in a small saucepan over medium-low heat and season well with salt and pepper. Cook, stirring, until warmed through.
5. Serve two chicken croquettes per person with the sauce and your choice of salad or vegetables.

Nutrition Info:
- 435 calories; 36 g protein; 27 g total fat; 7 g saturated fat; 10 g carbohydrates; 0 g fiber; 899 mg sodium

Lemon Thyme Chicken

Servings:3 | Cooking Time:x

Ingredients:
- 4 chicken thighs and 4 drumsticks (about 2 1/2 pounds)
- 3 medium lemons
- Zest of 1 medium lemon
- 1 tablespoon butter
- 1/4 teaspoon sea salt
- 1/2 teaspoon freshly ground black pepper
- 2 tablespoons fresh thyme leaves
- 6 basil leaves, torn

Directions:
1. Preheat oven to 375°F.
2. Add chicken to a large bowl. Slice lemons in half and juice into bowl.
3. Add lemon zest, butter, salt, pepper, and thyme; toss well with your hands. Place chicken in a 9" × 13" baking dish.
4. Bake 35–40 minutes, basting every 10 minutes. Skin should get crispy and meat should be cooked through.
5. Garnish with basil leaves.

Nutrition Info:
- Calories: 90,Fat: 5g,Protein: 6g,Sodium: 219mg,Carbohydrates: 9.

Pork And Fennel Meatballs

Servings:24 | Cooking Time:x

Ingredients:
- 1 pound lean ground pork
- 2 tablespoons roughly chopped fresh flat-leaf parsley
- 3 tablespoons gluten-free panko bread crumbs
- 1 large egg
- 1/8 teaspoon wheat-free asafetida powder
- 1/4 teaspoon salt
- 1/2 teaspoon freshly ground black pepper
- 1 1/2 tablespoons olive oil
- 2 teaspoons fennel seeds

Directions:
1. In a mixing bowl, combine pork, parsley, bread crumbs, egg, asafetida, salt, and pepper. Stir to combine or mix well with hands. Shape into 1" meatballs.
2. In a medium skillet, heat oil over medium heat and toast fennel seeds until fragrant, about 4 minutes. Add meatballs to pan.
3. Brown meatballs on all sides, cooking about 4–5 minutes per side, 20 minutes total. Meatballs are cooked through when no longer pink inside.

Nutrition Info:
- Calories: 64, Fat: 5g, Protein: 4g, Sodium: 47mg, Carbohydrates: 1.

Pan-fried Chicken With Brown Butter–sage Sauce

Servings:4 | Cooking Time:x

Ingredients:
- 2 teaspoons garlic-infused olive oil
- 2 teaspoons olive oil
- 1 tablespoon plus 1 teaspoon fresh lemon juice
- Salt and freshly ground black pepper
- Four 6-ounce (170 g) boneless, skinless chicken breasts
- 5 tablespoons (75 g) salted butter
- 2 garlic cloves, peeled and halved
- 20 sage leaves
- Shaved pecorino, for garnish
- Green salad or vegetables, for serving

Directions:
1. Combine the garlic-infused oil, olive oil, lemon juice, salt, and pepper in a bowl. Add the chicken breasts and toss to coat. Cover and refrigerate for 3 to 4 hours or overnight.
2. Melt 1 tablespoon of the butter in a large frying pan over medium-low heat. Add the chicken breasts and cook for 4 to 5 minutes on each side, until just cooked and golden brown.
3. Meanwhile, melt the remaining 4 tablespoons butter in a small frying pan and cook the garlic until golden brown. Remove the garlic from the pan and discard. Add the sage leaves to the butter and cook until the butter is golden brown.
4. Spoon the brown butter sauce over the chicken and garnish with the shaved pecorino. Serve with your choice of salad or vegetables.

Nutrition Info:
- 334 calories; 39 g protein; 19 g total fat; 10 g saturated fat; 1 g carbohydrates; 0 g fiber; 401 mg sodium

Garden Veggie Dip Burgers

Servings:4 | Cooking Time:x

Ingredients:
- 2 tablespoons light sour cream
- 1 large carrot, peeled and diced
- 1/2 medium red bell pepper, seeded and diced
- 1/2 cup packed baby spinach leaves, chopped
- 1 teaspoon sea salt
- 1 pound lean ground beef

Directions:
1. In a food processor, blend sour cream, carrot, pepper, spinach, and salt until creamy.
2. In a large bowl, add vegetable mixture to ground beef and mix to combine. Make 4 patties. Refrigerate patties for 12–24 hours before grilling.
3. Heat a charcoal or gas grill to 350°F. Cook patties on grill to an internal temperature of 160°F, about 5 minutes per side.

Nutrition Info:
- Calories: 177, Fat: 7g, Protein: 25g, Sodium: 680mg, Carbohydrates: 3.

Chicken Tenders

Servings:4 | Cooking Time: 15 Minutes

Ingredients:
- 1 cup gluten-free bread crumbs
- 1 teaspoon dried thyme
- ½ teaspoon sea salt
- ⅛ teaspoon freshly ground black pepper
- 2 eggs, beaten
- 1 tablespoon Dijon mustard
- 1 pound boneless skinless chicken breast, cut into strips

Directions:
1. Preheat the oven to 425°F.
2. In a medium bowl, mix the bread crumbs, thyme, salt, and pepper.
3. In a small bowl, whisk the eggs and mustard.
4. Dip the chicken strips into the egg mixture and into the bread crumb mixture to coat. Place them on a nonstick rimmed baking sheet.
5. Bake for 15 to 20 minutes, until the breading is golden and the juices run clear.

Nutrition Info:
- Calories:183; Total Fat: 5g; Saturated Fat: 2g; Carbohydrates: 20g; Fiber: 2g; Sodium: 526mg; Protein: 13g

Chicken Parmigiana

Servings: 4 | Cooking Time: x

Ingredients:
- One 14.5-ounce (425 g) can crushed tomatoes
- 2 heaping tablespoons chopped flat-leaf parsley
- 1 teaspoon sweet paprika
- 2 teaspoons sugar
- ½ cup (80 g) sliced black olives
- ½ cup (75 g) cornstarch
- 2 large eggs
- 1 cup (120 g) dried gluten-free, soy-free bread crumbs*
- Salt and freshly ground black pepper
- Four 6-ounce (170 g) boneless, skinless chicken breasts
- 1 tablespoon olive oil
- ⅔ cup (80 g) grated reduced-fat Parmesan or cheddar
- Green salad or vegetables, for serving

Directions:
1. Preheat the oven to 350°F (180°C).
2. To make the sauce, combine the tomatoes, parsley, paprika, sugar, and olives in a small frying pan and cook over medium-low heat for 15 minutes, stirring occasionally.
3. Set out three shallow bowls and fill one with the cornstarch, one with the eggs, and one with the bread crumbs mixed with the salt and pepper. Beat the eggs lightly. Coat the chicken breasts in the cornstarch, shaking off any excess, then dip in the egg, and finally toss in the bread crumbs until well coated.
4. Heat the olive oil in a large frying pan over medium-low heat. Add the chicken and cook for 3 to 4 minutes on each side, until golden brown and cooked through.
5. Place the chicken breasts in a baking dish, spoon the sauce over them, and top with the cheddar. Cover and bake for 15 minutes, or until the cheese is golden and melted.
6. Serve with your choice of salad or vegetables.

Nutrition Info:
- 516 calories; 50 g protein; 16 g total fat; 5 g saturated fat; 37 g carbohydrates; 2 g fiber; 805 mg sodium

Stuffed Rolled Roast Beef With Popovers And Gravy

Servings: 8 | Cooking Time: x

Ingredients:
- ½ cup (65 g) superfine white rice flour
- ⅓ cup (50 g) cornstarch
- 1 teaspoon salt
- 2 large eggs
- ½ cup (125 ml) skim milk, lactose-free milk, or suitable plant-based milk
- ⅔ cup (80 g) dried gluten-free, soy-free bread crumbs*
- 1 large egg
- ¼ cup (60 ml) gluten-free whole grain mustard
- 3 to 4 heaping tablespoons roughly chopped flat-leaf parsley
- 1 heaping tablespoon tomato paste or puree
- ¼ teaspoon salt
- ¼ teaspoon freshly ground black pepper
- 2 teaspoons paprika
- 2 pounds 10 ounces (1.2 kg) beef tenderloin
- 1 tablespoon olive oil
- 2 teaspoons salt
- 2 tablespoons vegetable oil
- About 1 cup (250 ml) boiling water
- ¼ cup (85 g) gluten-free, onion-free gravy mix*
- Roasted vegetables, for serving

Directions:
1. Preheat the oven to 400°F (200°C).
2. To make the popovers, sift the rice flour, cornstarch, and salt three times into a large bowl (or whisk in the bowl until well combined). Make a well in the middle and add the eggs and one third of the milk. Using a wooden spoon, mix the batter from the center out—first mixing the eggs and milk together, and then gradually working in the flour from the sides. Beat the batter until smooth and shiny. Stir in the remaining milk and let stand for 1 hour.
3. To make the stuffing, combine all the ingredients in a bowl. Set aside.
4. Place the beef on a cutting board and slice horizontally through the thickest part to open out the meat like a book. Press the stuffing along the center. Carefully roll up the beef to enclose the stuffing and secure with kitchen string at ¾-inch (2 cm) intervals.
5. Place the rolled beef in a metal baking dish, seam-side down, brush with the olive oil, and sprinkle with the salt. Roast for 40 to 45 minutes for medium-rare, or until your desired doneness. Remove from the oven and increase the oven temperature to 425°F (220°C). Transfer the beef to a cutting board and let rest, covered loosely with foil, while you make the popovers.
6. To make the popovers, put ½ teaspoon of vegetable oil into each cup of a 12-cup muffin pan. Place on the top shelf of the oven for 5 minutes to heat the oil. Carefully pour the batter into each cup. Reduce the heat to 375°F (190°C) and bake for 6 to 8 minutes, until the popovers are risen and golden brown.
7. To make the gravy, combine the pan juices with enough boiling water to equal 1 cup (250 ml) liquid. Return to the baking dish and whisk in the gravy mix. Cook over medium heat, whisking constantly, until thickened and well combined.
8. Remove the string from the beef and slice carefully so you don't disturb the stuffing. Serve with the popovers, gravy, and your choice of roasted vegetables.

Nutrition Info:
- 578 calories; 31 g protein; 40 g total fat; 15 g saturated fat; 22 g carbohydrates; 0 g fiber; 1205 mg sodium

Chicken Pockets

Servings: 4 | Cooking Time: x

Ingredients:
- Four 6-ounce (170 g) boneless, skinless chicken breasts
- ⅔ cup (100 g) sun-dried tomatoes, drained (if packed in oil) and finely chopped
- 1 cup (150 g) cooked white rice
- 3½ ounces (100 g) feta, finely diced (about ⅔ cup)
- 1 heaping tablespoon finely grated lemon zest
- 1 large egg white
- 2 heaping tablespoons fresh oregano
- Salt and freshly ground black pepper
- 2 teaspoons garlic-infused olive oil
- 3 tablespoons olive oil
- 1 teaspoon fresh oregano
- 1 teaspoon finely grated lemon zest
- 6 ounces (170 g) mashed sweet potato (from about 1 small sweet potato)
- 1 cup (150 g) cooked white rice
- 1 teaspoon ground cumin
- 1 large egg white
- Salt and freshly ground black pepper
- 2 teaspoons garlic-infused olive oil
- 3 tablespoons olive oil
- 1 teaspoon ground cumin
- 2 heaping tablespoons Basil Pesto
- 1 cup (150 g) cooked white rice
- 1 large egg white
- Salt and freshly ground black pepper
- 2 teaspoons garlic-infused olive oil
- 3 tablespoons olive oil
- 1 teaspoon Basil Pesto
- Small basil leaves, for garnish (optional)
- Green salad or vegetables, for serving

Directions:
1. Preheat the oven to 350°F (180°C).
2. Using a small sharp knife, insert the blade into the middle of the chicken breast and work to form a pocket (you want to cut to about ⅓ inch/1 cm from the internal edge).
3. Combine all the ingredients for your choice of filling in a medium bowl and mix well.
4. Spoon the filling into the chicken pockets, pressing it in firmly and making sure it is evenly spread. Seal the ends with a toothpick.
5. Place the chicken breasts on a baking sheet. Whisk together all the ingredients for your choice of basting liquid and brush it over the chicken. Bake for 15 minutes, or until golden brown, then cover with foil and bake for 5 to 10 minutes more, until cooked through (no longer pink inside). Let rest for 5 to 10 minutes.
6. Cut into thick slices, garnish with basil leaves (if desired), and serve with your choice of salad or vegetables.

Nutrition Info:
- 393 calories; 42 g protein; 19 g total fat; 3 g saturated fat; 12 g carbohydrates; 0 g fiber; 309 mg sodium

Lamb And Vegetable Pilaf

Servings: 4 | Cooking Time: x

Ingredients:
- 2 tablespoons olive oil
- 2 teaspoons garlic-infused olive oil
- 2½ teaspoons grated ginger
- 2 teaspoons ground cinnamon
- 6 whole cloves
- ½ teaspoon cayenne pepper
- 2 teaspoons ground cumin
- 1¼ pounds (500 g) boneless lamb loin, sliced
- 1½ cups (300 g) white basmati rice
- 1 small sweet potato, chopped
- 2½ cups (625 ml) gluten-free, onion-free beef or vegetable stock*
- ⅔ cup (65 g) slivered almonds
- 1 large eggplant, trimmed and sliced
- 2 medium zucchini, halved lengthwise and thickly sliced
- Salt and freshly ground black pepper
- ¼ cup (5 g) roughly chopped cilantro
- 3 tablespoons roughly chopped flat-leaf parsley

Directions:
1. Heat 1 tablespoon plus 2 teaspoons of the olive oil and the 2 teaspoons garlic-infused oil in a large saucepan or Dutch oven over medium heat. Add the ginger, cinnamon, cloves, cayenne, and cumin and cook for 1 to 2 minutes, until fragrant. Add the lamb and toss until browned.
2. Add the rice, sweet potato, and eggplant to the pan and cook, stirring, for 2 to 3 minutes, until the rice is well coated in the spiced oil. Pour in the stock and bring to a boil, then reduce the heat to low and simmer, covered, for 10 minutes.
3. Meanwhile, heat the remaining 1 teaspoon of olive oil in a small frying pan over medium heat. Add the almonds and cook, stirring, until golden. Drain on paper towels.
4. Add the zucchini to the rice mixture and cook for 5 minutes more, or until all the liquid has been absorbed and the rice is tender. Remove and discard the whole cloves. Season with salt and pepper, then stir in the almonds, cilantro, and parsley. Serve hot.

Nutrition Info:
- 630 calories; 24 g protein; 34 g total fat; 11 g saturated fat; 54 g carbohydrates; 7 g fiber; 318 mg sodium

Chicken And Rice With Peanut Sauce

Servings:4 | Cooking Time: 10 Minutes

Ingredients:
- 2 tablespoons Garlic Oil
- 1 pound boneless skinless chicken thigh meat, cut into strips
- ½ cup sugar-free natural peanut butter
- ½ cup coconut milk
- 2 tablespoons gluten-free soy sauce
- 1 tablespoon peeled and grated fresh ginger
- Juice of 1 lime
- 2 cups cooked brown rice

Directions:
1. In a large nonstick skillet over medium-high heat, heat the garlic oil until it shimmers.
2. Add the chicken and cook for about 6 minutes, stirring occasionally, until browned.
3. In a small bowl, whisk the peanut butter, coconut milk, soy sauce, ginger, and lime juice. Add this to the chicken.
4. Mix in the rice. Cook for 3 minutes more, stirring.

Nutrition Info:
- Calories:718; Total Fat: 40g; Saturated Fat: 13g; Carbohydrates: 46g; Fiber: 5g; Sodium: 757mg; Protein: 46g

Pecan-crusted Maple-mustard Salmon

Servings:4 | Cooking Time: 12 Minutes

Ingredients:
- Cooking spray
- 2 tablespoons Dijon mustard
- 2 tablespoons maple syrup
- 4 (6-ounce) salmon fillets
- ½ cup finely chopped pecans

Directions:
1. Preheat the oven to 425°F.
2. Coat a baking dish with cooking spray. In a small bowl, stir together the mustard and maple syrup. Arrange the salmon fillets in a single layer in the baking dish. Spread the mustard–maple syrup mixture over the tops of the fillets. Sprinkle the pecans on top, pressing them into the mustard mixture.
3. Bake in the preheated oven for about 12 minutes, until the salmon is cooked through and flakes easily with a fork. Serve immediately.

Nutrition Info:
- Calories: 305; Protein: 34g; Total Fat: 16g; Saturated Fat: 2g; Carbohydrates: 8g; Fiber: 1g; Sodium: 165mg;

Pumpkin Maple Roast Chicken

Servings:4 | Cooking Time:x

Ingredients:
- 1 1/2 tablespoons butter
- 1 tablespoon canned pumpkin
- 1 tablespoon pure maple syrup
- 1 teaspoon ground cinnamon
- 1 teaspoon dried thyme
- 1/2 teaspoon sea salt
- 1/4 teaspoon freshly ground black pepper
- 1 (4-pound) whole chicken

Directions:
1. Preheat oven to 375°F.
2. Melt butter in a small saucepan. Stir in pumpkin, maple syrup, cinnamon, thyme, salt, and pepper. Refrigerate 10 minutes.
3. Cut small slit under skin on both sides of chicken breast and under legs. Once the pumpkin mixture is cool, generously rub it under skin and all over the top of skin. Place chicken, breast side up, on the rack of a roasting pan. Roast 50–60 minutes or until a meat thermometer registers 165°F at thickest part of thigh.
4. Tent with foil and let rest 5 minutes before carving.

Nutrition Info:
- Calories: 588,Fat: 18g,Protein: 96g,Sodium: 641mg,Carbohydrates: 4.

Chimichurri Chicken Drumsticks

Servings:4 | Cooking Time: 30 Minutes

Ingredients:
- 8 chicken drumsticks
- 1 cup Chimichurri Sauce, divided

Directions:
1. In a gallon-size zip-top bag, combine the drumsticks with ½ cup chimichurri sauce. Seal the bag and shake to coat. Refrigerate for 8 hours.
2. Preheat the oven to 375°F.
3. Line a rimmed baking sheet with parchment paper.
4. Remove the drumsticks from the bag, pat the marinade off with a paper towel (a little will be left, which is okay), and place them on the prepared baking sheet. Bake for about 30 minutes, or until the juices run clear.
5. Serve with the remaining ½ cup chimichurri sauce on the side.

Nutrition Info:
- Calories:401; Total Fat: 11g; Saturated Fat: 3g; Carbohydrates: 39g; Fiber: 3g; Sodium: 968mg; Protein: 35g

Crispy Baked Chicken With Gravy

Servings: 4 | Cooking Time: x

Ingredients:
- 2 cups brown rice
- 4 cups water
- 2 1/2 pounds boneless, skinless chicken breasts
- 1 cup gluten-free panko bread crumbs
- 4 tablespoons olive oil, divided
- 2 tablespoons minced fresh flat-leaf parsley
- 1/4 cup Dijon mustard
- 2 tablespoons water
- 1/4 teaspoon salt, divided
- 1/2 teaspoon freshly ground black pepper, divided
- 6 tablespoons butter
- 1/2 cup plus 6 tablespoons gluten-free all-purpose flour
- 1 cup lactose-free milk
- 1 cup chicken stock
- 1/4 teaspoon dried thyme

Directions:
1. Place rice in a medium saucepan with water. Bring to a boil, reduce heat to low, and cover; simmer 20 minutes. Rice should be tender. Remove from heat, stir, and keep covered. Set aside.
2. Preheat oven to 400°F. Line a baking sheet with aluminum foil. Place a rack over pan and spray rack with nonstick cooking spray.
3. Using a meat tenderizer, pound each chicken breast to a 1/4" thickness. Set aside.
4. In a shallow dish, combine bread crumbs, 2 tablespoons olive oil, and parsley. In a separate shallow dish, combine mustard, water, 1/8 teaspoon salt, and 1/4 teaspoon pepper, and remaining olive oil.
5. Coat each chicken breast with mustard mixture; dredge each in bread crumb mixture. Place on prepared rack in pan.
6. Bake 25–30 minutes or until chicken is golden brown. About 15–20 minutes into baking chicken, prepare gravy.
7. For gravy: Over medium heat, melt butter in a medium saucepan and whisk in flour to make a roux (a mixture of fat and flour used in making sauces). Whisk constantly until bubbling and flour turns light brown in color. Gradually whisk in milk, stock, and thyme, and continue to stir. Add 1/8 teaspoon salt and 1/4 teaspoon pepper. Mixture should thicken after about 5 minutes.
8. Divide rice onto 4 plates. Place chicken breasts on rice and spoon gravy on top. Serve immediately.

Nutrition Info:
- Calories: 765, Fat: 30g, Protein: 51g, Sodium: 573mg, Carbohydrates: 69.

Thai Sweet Chili Broiled Salmon

Servings: 4 | Cooking Time: 10 Minutes

Ingredients:
- 6 tablespoons homemade Thai Sweet Chili Sauce (here)
- 3 tablespoons gluten-free soy sauce
- 1 tablespoon finely grated fresh ginger
- 4 (6-ounce) salmon fillets
- 2 scallions (green part only), thinly sliced
- 1 tablespoon chopped fresh cilantro
- 1 1/2 teaspoons toasted sesame seeds

Directions:
1. In a large bowl, combine the chili sauce, soy sauce, and ginger, and mix well. Add the fish, turning until evenly coated. Cover the bowl and marinate fish in the refrigerator for 30 minutes.
2. To cook the fish, heat the broiler to high and line a rimmed baking sheet with foil.
3. Arrange the salmon fillets skin-side down on the prepared baking sheet. Brush some of the marinade over the fish, coating generously. Broil for about 8 to 10 minutes, until just cooked through. Serve immediately, garnished with scallions, cilantro, and sesame seeds.

Nutrition Info:
- Calories: 291; Protein: 34g; Total Fat: 11g; Saturated Fat: 2g; Carbohydrates: 13g; Fiber: 1g; Sodium: 812mg;

Spinach And Feta-stuffed Chicken Breast

Servings: 2 | Cooking Time: x

Ingredients:
- 1 tablespoon garlic-infused oil
- 8 ounces spinach
- 1/2 cup crumbled feta cheese
- 2 boneless, skinless chicken breasts, pounded to a 1/4" thickness
- 1 large egg, lightly beaten
- 1 cup gluten-free bread crumbs

Directions:
1. Preheat oven to 350°F.
2. Heat oil in a medium skillet over low heat; cook spinach until soft, about 2–3 minutes. Add feta, stir a few times, and remove from heat.
3. Lay spinach mixture onto each chicken breast. Wrap chicken breasts around mixture and secure with toothpicks.
4. Place egg in a shallow bowl. Place bread crumbs in a separate shallow bowl. Roll each breast in egg, tap off any excess, then roll in bread crumbs until well coated.
5. Place in an 8" × 8" casserole dish. Bake 30 minutes and serve.

Nutrition Info:
- Calories: 468, Fat: 17g, Protein: 46g, Sodium: 807mg, Carbohydrates: 30.

Italian-herbed Chicken Meatballs In Broth

Servings:4 | Cooking Time: 25 Minutes

Ingredients:
- FOR THE MEATBALLS
- Oil for preparing the baking sheet
- 1 pound ground chicken
- ¾ cup cooked rice
- ½ cup chopped fresh basil
- 1½ ounces freshly grated Parmesan cheese, plus more for garnish
- 1 tablespoon Garlic Oil (here)
- 1 egg, lightly beaten
- 1¼ teaspoons salt
- ½ teaspoon freshly ground black pepper
- FOR THE BROTH
- 1 tablespoon olive oil
- 1 tablespoon Garlic Oil (here)
- 1 large carrot, thinly sliced
- 5 cups homemade (onion- and garlic-free) chicken broth
- 4 cups baby spinach
- ½ cup chopped fresh basil

Directions:
1. Preheat the oven to 400°F.
2. Line a large, rimmed baking sheet with parchment paper lightly coated with oil.
3. In a large bowl, combine the chicken, rice, basil, cheese, Garlic Oil, egg, salt, and pepper, and mix well. Form the mixture into 1-inch balls and arrange them on the prepared baking sheet. Bake in the preheated oven for about 25 minutes, until the meatballs are browned and cooked through.
4. Meanwhile, make the broth. Heat the olive oil and Garlic Oil in a stockpot over medium-high heat. Add the carrots and cook, stirring, for 3 minutes, then add the broth and bring to a boil. Reduce the heat to low and simmer, uncovered, for about 10 minutes, until the carrots are tender. Stir in the spinach and basil, and cook just until wilted, for about 3 minutes.
5. To serve, place several meatballs in a serving bowl, and ladle the broth and vegetables over the top. Serve immediately, garnished with additional Parmesan cheese if desired.

Nutrition Info:
- Calories: 493; Protein: 48g; Total Fat: 17g; Saturated Fat: 5g; Carbohydrates: 33g; Fiber: 2g; Sodium: 1933mg;

Turkey Dijon

Servings:4 | Cooking Time: 15 Minutes

Ingredients:
- 2 tablespoons Garlic Oil
- 4 (4-ounce) turkey cutlets, pounded to ¼-inch thickness
- 2 tablespoons Dijon mustard
- 1 cup Low-FODMAP Poultry Broth
- 1 tablespoon cornstarch
- ½ teaspoon sea salt
- ⅛ teaspoon freshly ground black pepper

Directions:
1. In a large nonstick skillet over medium-high heat, heat the garlic oil until it shimmers.
2. Add the turkey and cook for about 4 minutes per side, until the juices run clear. Transfer the turkey to a plate and tent with aluminum foil to keep warm. Return the skillet to the heat.
3. In a small bowl, whisk the broth, cornstarch, salt, and pepper. Whisk this into the hot skillet and cook for 1 to 2 minutes, whisking until the sauce thickens.
4. Serve the turkey with the sauce spooned over the top.

Nutrition Info:
- Calories:270; Total Fat: 13g; Saturated Fat: 3g; Carbohydrates: 3g; Fiber: 0g; Sodium: 420mg; Protein: 34g

Easy Pan Chicken

Servings:4 | Cooking Time:x

Ingredients:
- 3 tablespoons whole-grain mustard
- 2 teaspoons dried oregano
- 1 teaspoon dried thyme
- 1 tablespoon unsalted butter, softened
- 2 teaspoons Dijon mustard
- 3 pounds bone-in chicken thighs and drumsticks, patted dry
- 1/2 teaspoon salt
- 1 teaspoon freshly ground black pepper
- 2/3 cup plain gluten-free bread crumbs
- 4 medium carrots, peeled and halved lengthwise
- 1 tablespoon garlic-infused olive oil

Directions:
1. Heat oven to 425°F.
2. In a small bowl, combine whole-grain mustard, oregano, thyme, butter, and Dijon mustard.
3. Season chicken with salt and pepper. Rub mustard-butter mixture all over chicken.
4. Place bread crumbs in a wide bowl and coat chicken evenly with bread crumbs.
5. Place carrots (cut side down) with chicken on a baking sheet and drizzle with olive oil.
6. Bake until chicken is golden and no longer pink, 35–40 minutes.

Nutrition Info:
- Calories: 564,Fat: 21g,Protein: 70g,Sodium: 733mg,Carbohydrates: 20.

Stuffed Peppers With Ground Turkey

Servings:3 | Cooking Time:x

Ingredients:
- 1 tablespoon olive oil
- 1 pound ground turkey
- 1 tablespoon garlic-infused oil, divided
- 1 cup roasted corn kernels
- 2 Roma tomatoes, chopped
- 2 tablespoons pine nuts
- 1 cup cooked brown rice
- 1/2 tablespoon chili powder
- 1/2 teaspoon ground cumin
- 1 teaspoon smoked paprika
- 3 tablespoons chopped fresh cilantro
- 3 large bell peppers: orange, yellow, and green; halved and seeded
- 2 tablespoons coconut oil
- 6 slices goat cheese
- 3 tablespoons Fiesta Salsa (see Chapter 13)

Directions:
1. Preheat oven to 375°F.
2. Heat 1 tablespoon olive oil in a large skillet over medium-high heat and cook ground turkey until browned.
3. Add 1/2 tablespoon garlic-infused oil to skillet along with corn, tomatoes, and pine nuts; stir and heat through.
4. Add brown rice and stir to combine. Stir in remaining 1/2 tablespoon oil, chili powder, cumin, paprika, and cilantro. Remove from heat.
5. Stuff halved peppers with brown rice mixture and brush outside of peppers with coconut oil. Place peppers in an 8" × 8" shallow baking dish.
6. Top each pepper with a slice of goat cheese. Loosely cover dish with foil.
7. Bake 30–40 minutes until peppers are tender. Garnish with salsa.

Nutrition Info:
- Calories: 700,Fat: 43g,Protein: 41g,Sodium: 364mg,Carbohydrates: 41.

Dijon-roasted Pork Tenderloin

Servings:8 | Cooking Time: 60 Minutes

Ingredients:
- 1 pork loin roast (about 4 pounds), trimmed of excess fat
- 1 teaspoon salt
- 1/2 teaspoon pepper
- 1/4 cup whole-grain Dijon mustard
- 1/4 cup brown sugar

Directions:
1. Preheat the oven to 425°F.
2. Season the roast all over with the salt and pepper, place it on a roasting rack in a roasting pan, and roast in the preheated oven for 30 minutes.
3. Brush the mustard over the entire roast, then sprinkle the brown sugar over it, pressing the sugar into the mustard.
4. Lower the oven heat to 375°F and continue roasting, basting now and then with the drippings, for about 30 minutes more, until a meat thermometer inserted into the center of the roast reads 145°F. Remove the roast from the oven, tent loosely with aluminum foil, and let rest for 10 minutes before slicing.
5. To serve, slice the roast into 1/2-inch-thick slices, and spoon a bit of the drippings over them.

Nutrition Info:
- Calories: 499; Protein: 65g; Total Fat: 22g; Saturated Fat: 8g; Carbohydrates: 5g; Fiber: 0g; Sodium: 604mg;

Asian-style Pork Meatballs

Servings:4 | Cooking Time: 40 Minutes

Ingredients:
- Oil for preparing the baking sheet
- 1 1/4 pounds ground pork
- 1/4 cup finely chopped fresh basil
- 1 tablespoon Garlic Oil (here)
- 2 scallions, green parts only, thinly sliced
- 1 tablespoon fish sauce
- 1 teaspoon onion- and garlic-free chili paste
- 1 tablespoon sugar
- 2 teaspoons cornstarch
- 1 teaspoon salt
- 1 teaspoon freshly ground black pepper

Directions:
1. Preheat the oven to 350°F.
2. Line a large, rimmed baking sheet with lightly oiled parchment paper. In a large bowl, combine the pork, basil, Garlic Oil, scallions, fish sauce, chili paste, sugar, cornstarch, salt, and pepper, and mix to combine. With wet hands, form the mixture into 2-inch balls. Place the meatballs on the prepared baking sheet as they are formed.
3. Bake the meatballs in the preheated oven for about 40 minutes, until they are browned and cooked through. Serve hot.

Nutrition Info:
- Calories: 232; Protein: 38g; Total Fat: 5g; Saturated Fat: 2g; Carbohydrates: 7g; Fiber: 0g; Sodium: 1027mg;

Fish With Thai Red Curry Sauce

Servings: 4 | Cooking Time: 30 Minutes

Ingredients:
- 1 tablespoon grapeseed oil
- ¼ cup Thai Red Curry Paste (here)
- 2½ cups coconut milk
- 2 tablespoons fish sauce
- 2 Kaffir lime leaves
- 1 sweet potato, peeled and diced
- 1 zucchini, diced
- 1 cup green beans, cut into 1-inch pieces
- 1½ pounds fish fillet
- ¼ cup crushed toasted peanuts
- ¼ cup chopped fresh cilantro

Directions:

1. Heat the oil in a large saucepan over medium-high heat. Add the curry paste and cook, stirring, for about 1 minute. Stir in the coconut milk, fish sauce, and lime leaves, and bring to a boil.
2. Add the sweet potato, reduce the heat to low, and simmer for 10 minutes. Stir in the zucchini and green beans, and continue to cook for about 10 minutes more, until the vegetables are tender.
3. Add the fish and cook for 7 to 9 minutes more, until the fish is cooked through. Serve hot, garnished with peanuts and cilantro.

Nutrition Info:
- Calories: 571; Protein: 23g; Total Fat: 35g; Saturated Fat: 7g; Carbohydrates: 44g; Fiber: 5g; Sodium: 2261mg;

Beef Stir-fry With Chinese Broccoli And Green Beans

Servings: 4 | Cooking Time: x

Ingredients:
- 1 heaping tablespoon grated ginger
- 2 teaspoons garlic-infused olive oil
- 2 teaspoons olive oil
- ¼ cup (60 ml) sesame oil
- 1 pound (450 g) beef sirloin or top round steak, very thinly sliced
- 1 bunch Chinese broccoli, cut into 1-inch (3 cm) lengths
- 7 ounces (200 g) green beans, trimmed (1¾ cups)
- 1 cup (80 g) bean sprouts
- 1 tablespoon gluten-free, onion-free, garlic-free oyster sauce
- ¼ teaspoon cayenne pepper
- Steamed rice or prepared rice noodles, for serving

Directions:

1. Combine the ginger, garlic-infused oil, olive oil, and 2 tablespoons of the sesame oil in a bowl. Add the beef and toss to coat. Cover and refrigerate for 2 to 3 hours.
2. Heat the remaining 2 tablespoons of sesame oil in a wok over medium-high heat. Add the beef and cook for 2 minutes, or until lightly browned. Add the Chinese broccoli, green beans, and bean sprouts and stir-fry for 2 to 4 minutes, until the ingredients are tender. Pour in the oyster sauce and cayenne pepper and stir-fry for 1 to 2 minutes, until the sauce is warmed through and the beef and vegetables are coated.
3. Serve over rice or rice noodles.

Nutrition Info:
- 437 calories; 24 g protein; 34 g total fat; 6 g saturated fat; 7 g carbohydrates; 3 g fiber; 92 mg sodium

Soy-infused Roast Chicken

Servings: 4 | Cooking Time: x

Ingredients:
- ½ cup (125 ml) gluten-free soy sauce
- 2 tablespoons plus 2 teaspoons sesame oil
- 2 heaping tablespoons light brown sugar
- 2 teaspoons grated ginger
- 3 star anise (or 2 teaspoons ground star anise)
- ½ teaspoon ground cinnamon
- One 4-pound (1.8 kg) whole chicken, excess fat removed
- 2 cups (500 ml) gluten-free, onion-free chicken stock*
- Vegetables, for serving

Directions:

1. Combine the soy sauce, sesame oil, brown sugar, ginger, star anise, and cinnamon in a bowl and stir until the sugar has dissolved. Place the chicken, breast up, in a baking dish. Pour the marinade over it and use a pastry brush to ensure the entire chicken is well coated. Cover and refrigerate for 3 to 4 hours, brushing the chicken with the marinade every 1 to 2 hours.
2. Preheat the oven to 350°F (180°C).
3. Uncover the chicken, pour the stock into the baking dish, and roast for 30 minutes. Cover loosely with foil and roast for 20 to 30 minutes more, until the juices run clear when you piece the chicken with a toothpick in the thickest part of the thigh. Let rest for a few minutes before carving.
4. Serve with the pan juices and your choice of vegetables.

Nutrition Info:
- 304 calories; 40 g protein; 12 g total fat; 2 g saturated fat; 6 g carbohydrates; 0 g fiber; 1485 mg sodium

Snapper With Tropical Salsa

Servings:4 | Cooking Time: 8 Minutes

Ingredients:
- 2 tablespoons extra-virgin olive oil
- 1 pound snapper, quartered
- 1 teaspoon sea salt, divided
- ⅛ teaspoon freshly ground black pepper
- 1 papaya, chopped
- 1 cup chopped pineapple
- 1 jalapeño pepper, seeded and minced
- 1 tablespoon chopped fresh cilantro leaves
- Juice of 1 lime

Directions:
1. In a large nonstick skillet over medium-high heat, heat the olive oil until it shimmers.
2. Season the snapper with ½ teaspoon salt and the pepper. Add it to the skillet and cook for about 4 minutes per side, until the fish is opaque.
3. In a medium bowl, gently stir together the papaya, pineapple, jalapeño, cilantro, lime juice, and remaining ½ teaspoon salt.
4. Serve the salsa on top of the snapper.

Nutrition Info:
- Calories:236; Total Fat: 8g; Saturated Fat: 1g; Carbohydrates: 14g; Fiber: 2g; Sodium: 565mg; Protein: 27g

Polenta-crusted Chicken

Servings:2 | Cooking Time:x

Ingredients:
- 1 large egg
- 1/2 teaspoon salt, divided
- 1/2 teaspoon freshly ground black pepper, divided
- 1/4 cup gluten-free all-purpose flour
- 1/4 cup quick-cooking polenta
- 1 teaspoon dried oregano
- 1 teaspoon dried thyme
- 3/4 pound boneless, skinless chicken breasts
- 1/4 cup safflower oil
- 1/4 cup olive oil

Directions:
1. In a shallow bowl, beat egg with 1/4 teaspoon each of salt and pepper. In another shallow bowl, whisk together flour, polenta, oregano, thyme, and 1/4 teaspoon each of salt and pepper.
2. Dip chicken in egg, tapping off any excess, then dredge in polenta mixture.
3. Heat safflower oil and olive oil in a 6" nonstick skillet over medium heat.
4. Cook chicken in batches until golden brown, 4–6 minutes on one side and 2 minutes on other side.

Nutrition Info:
- Calories: 383,Fat: 31g,Protein: 20g,Sodium: 410mg,Carbohydrates: 7.

Quick Meatloaf Patties

Servings:4 | Cooking Time: 10 Minutes

Ingredients:
- 1 pound ground beef
- ½ cup gluten-free bread crumbs
- 1 egg, beaten
- 1 tablespoon Dijon mustard
- 1 tablespoon Worcestershire sauce
- 1 teaspoon dried thyme
- 1 teaspoon sea salt
- ⅛ teaspoon freshly ground black pepper
- 2 tablespoons extra-virgin olive oil

Directions:
1. In a large bowl, combine the ground beef, bread crumbs, egg, mustard, Worcestershire sauce, thyme, salt, and pepper. Mix well. Form the meat mixture into 4 patties.
2. In a large nonstick skillet over medium-high heat, heat the olive oil until it shimmers.
3. Add the patties and cook for about 5 minutes per side, until browned on both sides.

Nutrition Info:
- Calories:295; Total Fat: 15g; Saturated Fat: 4g; Carbohydrates: 2g; Fiber: 0g; Sodium: 644mg; Protein: 36g

Lemon-pepper Shrimp

Servings:4 | Cooking Time: 8 Minutes

Ingredients:
- 2 tablespoons Garlic Oil
- 1 pound medium shrimp, shelled and deveined
- Juice of 2 lemons
- ½ teaspoon sea salt
- ½ teaspoon freshly ground black pepper

Directions:
1. In a large nonstick skillet over medium-high heat, heat the garlic oil until it shimmers.
2. Add the shrimp. Cook for about 5 minutes, stirring occasionally, until it is pink.
3. Squeeze in the lemon juice, then add the salt and pepper. Simmer for 3 minutes more.

Nutrition Info:
- Calories:119; Total Fat: 2g; Saturated Fat: 0g; Carbohydrates: 2g; Fiber: 0g; Sodium: 494mg; Protein: 25g

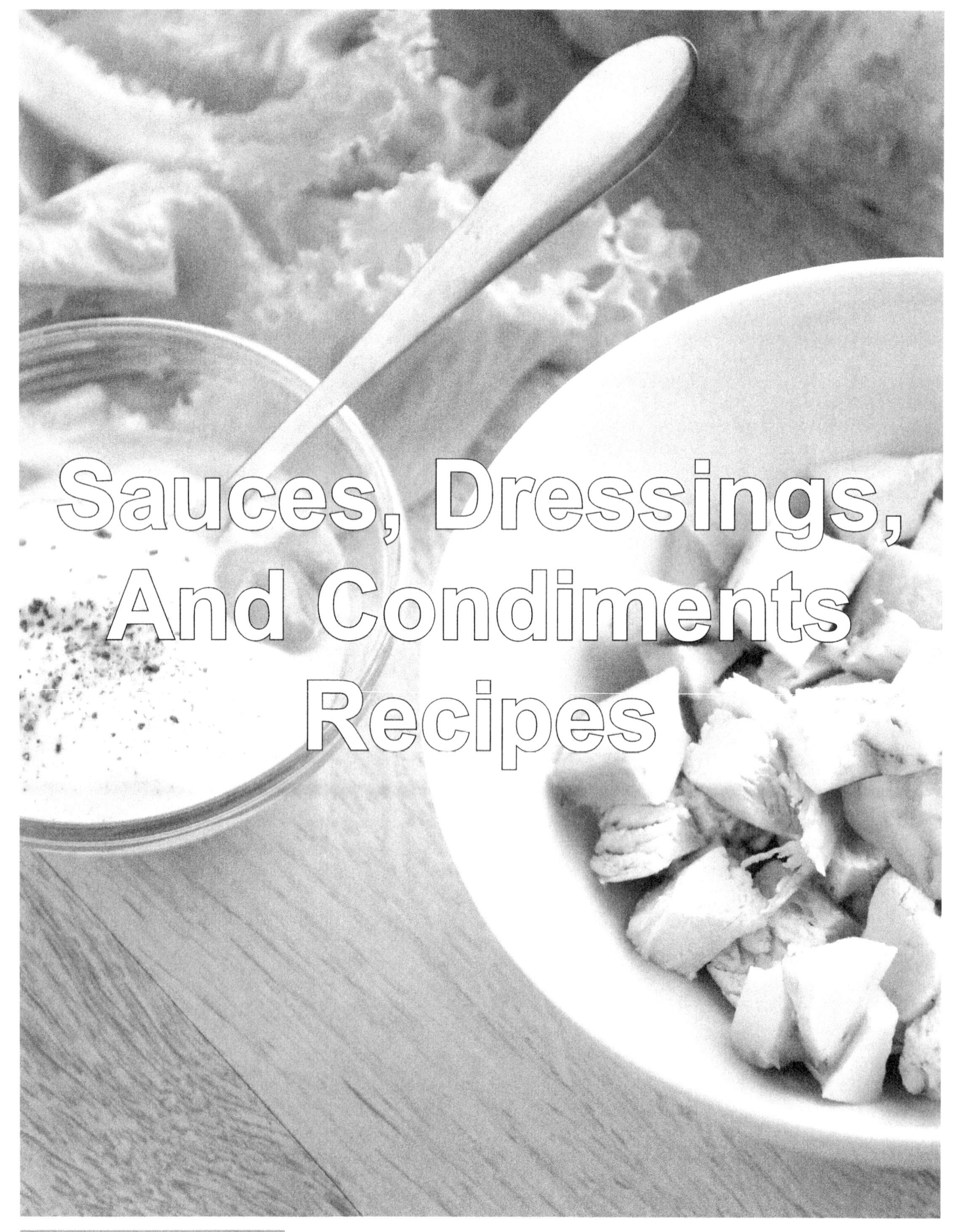

Sauces, Dressings, And Condiments Recipes

Sauces, Dressings, And Condiments Recipes

Luscious Hot Fudge Sauce

Servings: 2 | Cooking Time: 5 Minutes

Ingredients:
- ⅔ cup full-fat coconut milk
- ½ cup granulated sugar
- ⅓ cup brown sugar
- ¼ cup unsweetened cocoa powder
- ¼ teaspoon salt
- 6 ounces bittersweet chocolate (dairy-free and gluten-free), chopped, divided
- 2 tablespoons coconut oil
- 1 teaspoon vanilla extract

Directions:
1. In a medium saucepan combine the coconut milk, sugars, cocoa powder, salt, and half of the chocolate, and bring to a boil. Reduce the heat to low and simmer, stirring occasionally, for 5 minutes.
2. Remove the pan from the heat and whisk in the remaining chocolate along with the coconut oil and vanilla. Stir until smooth.
3. Let cool for 15 to 20 minutes before serving. Serve warm or store in a covered container in the refrigerator for up to 2 weeks.

Nutrition Info:
- Calories: 135; Protein: 2g; Total Fat: 8g; Saturated Fat: 6g; Carbohydrates: 17g; Fiber: 1g; Sodium: 48mg;

Low-fodmap Poultry Broth Or Meat Broth

Servings: 8 | Cooking Time: 3 To 8 Hours

Ingredients:
- 3 pounds meaty bones
- 3 carrots, roughly chopped
- 2 leeks, green parts only, roughly chopped
- 8 peppercorns
- 1 fresh thyme sprig

Directions:
1. In a large stockpot or slow cooker, combine the bones, carrots, leeks, peppercorns, and thyme.
2. Fill the pot about ¾ full, with enough water to cover the ingredients.
3. If using a stockpot: Place the pot over medium-low heat and bring the liquid to a simmer.
4. Simmer for 3 hours.
5. If using a slow cooker: Cover the cooker, set the temperature to low, and cook for 8 hours.
6. Strain and discard the solids.
7. Refrigerate the broth overnight. Skim the fat from the surface and discard.
8. Refrigerate or freeze the stock in 1-cup servings. The broth will keep in the refrigerator for about 5 days or in the freezer for up to 12 months.

Nutrition Info:
- Calories:Calories: 15; Total Fat: 0g; Saturated Fat: 0g; Carbohydrates: 1.5g; Fiber: 0g; Sodium: 60mg; Protein: 1.5g

Pumpkin Maple Glaze

Servings: 1 | Cooking Time: x

Ingredients:
- 2 tablespoons butter
- 1/4 cup hulled pumpkin seeds
- 1/8 teaspoon sea salt
- 3 tablespoons pure maple syrup, divided
- 1 tablespoon Dijon mustard

Directions:
1. Melt butter in a small saucepan over medium heat and set aside.
2. Preheat broiler. Spread pumpkin seeds on a lined baking sheet. Drizzle 1 tablespoon melted butter over pumpkin seeds. Sprinkle on salt. Toss seeds to coat. Broil 1–2 minutes or until seeds start to brown lightly. Remove from oven. Move seeds to serving dish and mix in 1 tablespoon maple syrup.
3. Return saucepan that contains the remaining tablespoon butter to cooktop. Over medium heat, add remaining maple syrup and mustard. Bring just to a boil, then lower heat and simmer, uncovered, 1–2 minutes more to thicken.
4. The glaze and roasted seeds can be used to top any roasted poultry.

Nutrition Info:
- Calories: 71,Fat: 5g,Protein: 1g,Sodium: 60mg,Carbohydrates: 6.

Tomato Paste

Servings: 1 | Cooking Time: x

Ingredients:
- 1 1/2 cups Tomato Purée (see recipe in this chapter)

Directions:
1. Preheat oven to 300°F. Pour purée into an ovenproof skillet.
2. Cook, uncovered, for about 2 hours, stirring every 20 minutes, until a paste consistency is formed.
3. Cool completely.

Nutrition Info:
- Calories: 22,Fat: 0g,Protein: 1g,Sodium: 475mg,Carbohydrates: 5.

Tahini Dressing

Servings: 3 | Cooking Time: x

Ingredients:
- 1/4 cup tahini
- 1/4 cup water
- 2 tablespoons fresh lemon juice
- 1 tablespoon maple syrup
- 1/4 teaspoon pink Himalayan salt
- 1/4 teaspoon freshly ground black pepper

Directions:
1. Combine all ingredients in a blender or food processor. Store in an air-tight container at room temperature for 1–2 weeks.

Nutrition Info:
- Calories: 70, Fat: 5g, Protein: 2g, Sodium: 111mg, Carbohydrates: 5.

Thai Red Curry Paste

Servings: 1 | Cooking Time: 1 Minute

Ingredients:
- 6 dry red chiles
- 1 teaspoon ground cumin
- 1 teaspoon ground coriander
- 1 teaspoon paprika
- 3-inch piece fresh ginger
- 2 (6-inch) pieces fresh lemongrass
- 2 tablespoons chopped fresh cilantro
- 2 teaspoons shrimp paste
- 2 Kaffir lime leaves
- ¼ teaspoon salt

Directions:
1. Place the chiles in a heatproof bowl and cover them with boiling water. Let soak for 15 minutes, then drain.
2. Heat a medium skillet over medium-high heat, add the cumin, coriander, and paprika, and cook, stirring, for about 1 minute, until fragrant. Transfer the spices to a food processor.
3. Add the ginger, lemongrass, cilantro, shrimp paste, lime leaves, and salt to the food processor, along with the drained chiles. Process to a smooth paste.
4. Refrigerate in a sealed container for up to a week, or freeze for up to 3 months.

Nutrition Info:
- Calories: 23; Protein: 1g; Total Fat: 0g; Saturated Fat: 0g; Carbohydrates: 5g; Fiber: 1g; Sodium: 193mg;

Basic Mayonnaise

Servings: 2 | Cooking Time: x

Ingredients:
- 2 large eggs
- 2 tablespoons Dijon mustard
- 1 1/3 cups safflower or sunflower oil
- 2 tablespoons freshly squeezed lemon juice
- 1/4 teaspoon salt
- 1/4 teaspoon freshly ground black pepper

Directions:
1. Use a food processor fitted with a blade attachment to combine eggs and mustard. Process until evenly combined.
2. Keep food processor running and add oil in a slow stream until completely combined.
3. Add lemon juice, salt, and pepper and pulse until smooth. If storing, place in a jar or container with a tight-fitting lid in refrigerator up to 3 days.

Nutrition Info:
- Calories: 86, Fat: 9g, Protein: 0g, Sodium: 34mg, Carbohydrates: 0.

Low-fodmap Worcestershire Sauce

Servings: 1 | Cooking Time: 20 Minutes

Ingredients:
- 2 cups rice vinegar
- 1 teaspoon balsamic vinegar
- ½ cup gluten-free soy sauce or tamari
- ¼ cup light-brown sugar
- 1 teaspoon ground ginger
- 1 teaspoon dry mustard
- 1 teaspoon cumin seeds
- ½ teaspoon fennel seeds
- ½ teaspoon ground cinnamon
- ½ teaspoon freshly ground black pepper

Directions:
1. In a medium saucepan, combine all of the ingredients and bring to a boil over medium-high heat. Reduce the heat to low and simmer, stirring occasionally, for 20 minutes or until the liquid has been reduced by about half.
2. Strain the mixture through a fine-meshed sieve, discarding the solids, and let cool to room temperature. Store in a covered container in the refrigerator for up to 3 months.

Nutrition Info:
- Calories: 21; Protein: 0g; Total Fat: 0g; Saturated Fat: 0g; Carbohydrates: 2g; Fiber: 0g; Sodium: 17mg;

Fiesta Salsa

Servings: 6 | Cooking Time: x

Ingredients:
- 1 (10-ounce) can diced tomatoes, drained
- 1 (14.5-ounce) can diced tomatoes with green chilies
- 1 tablespoon garlic-infused extra-virgin olive oil
- 1/4 cup chopped green onions, green part only
- 1/4 cup chopped fresh cilantro
- 1/4 cup chopped fresh flat-leaf parsley
- 1/8 teaspoon wheat-free asafetida powder
- 1/4 teaspoon ground cumin
- 1/4 teaspoon coriander
- 1/4 teaspoon dried oregano
- 1/4 teaspoon smoked paprika
- 1/4 teaspoon sea salt
- 1/2 teaspoon freshly ground black pepper
- Juice of 1 medium lime

Directions:
1. Add all ingredients to a medium serving bowl. Stir well to combine. Store in an airtight container in refrigerator 5–7 days.

Nutrition Info:
- Calories: 46, Fat: 3g, Protein: 1g, Sodium: 265mg, Carbohydrates: 6.

Ginger Sesame Salad Dressing

Servings: 1 | Cooking Time: x

Ingredients:
- 1/2 cup extra-virgin olive oil
- 1/4 cup rice wine vinegar
- 2 tablespoons gluten-free soy sauce (tamari)
- 2 tablespoons demerara sugar
- 1 teaspoon sesame oil
- 1" piece fresh gingerroot, minced

Directions:
1. Blend all ingredients in a blender or food processor until smooth. Dressing can be stored 1 week in refrigerator. Bring to room temperature before serving.

Nutrition Info:
- Calories: 141, Fat: 14g, Protein: 0g, Sodium: 226mg, Carbohydrates: 4.

Garlic-infused Oil

Servings: 1 | Cooking Time: x

Ingredients:
- 1 cup plus 1 teaspoon grapeseed oil
- 4 garlic cloves, peeled, slightly smashed

Directions:
1. Heat oil in a small saucepan over medium-low heat, add garlic, and sauté for 10 minutes, stirring often. Remove from heat and allow to completely cool. Remove and discard garlic, reserving oil.

Nutrition Info:
- Calories: 123, Fat: 14g, Protein: 0g, Sodium: 0mg, Carbohydrates: 0.

Sun-dried Tomato Pesto

Servings: 1 | Cooking Time: x

Ingredients:
- 2 tablespoons walnut oil
- 1/4 cup walnuts, toasted
- 1/4 cup sun-dried tomatoes
- 1 cup packed baby spinach leaves
- 1/2 teaspoon sea salt
- 1/4 cup freshly grated Parmesan cheese

Directions:
1. Add all ingredients to a food processor and blend to a pesto consistency.

Nutrition Info:
- Calories: 290, Fat: 27g, Protein: 9g, Sodium: 670mg, Carbohydrates: 7.

Egg-free Caesar Dressing

Servings: 1 | Cooking Time: None

Ingredients:
- 4 whole anchovy fillets
- 2 tablespoons Dijon mustard
- 1 tablespoon red-wine vinegar
- 1 teaspoon gluten-free soy sauce or coconut aminos
- Juice of ½ lemon
- ¼ teaspoon salt
- ¼ teaspoon freshly ground black pepper
- ¼ cup olive oil
- ¼ cup Garlic Oil (here)
- ¼ cup freshly grated Parmesan cheese

Directions:
1. In a blender or food processor, combine the anchovies, mustard, vinegar, soy sauce or coconut aminos, lemon juice, salt, and pepper. Pulse to chop the anchovies and combine well.
2. With the processor running, slowly add the olive oil and Garlic Oil in a thin stream. Process until the mixture is thickened. Add the cheese and pulse just to incorporate.
3. Serve immediately or store in a covered container in the refrigerator for up to a week.

Nutrition Info:
- Calories: 229; Protein: 18g; Total Fat: 17g; Saturated Fat: 4g; Carbohydrates: 2g; Fiber: 0g; Sodium: 3632mg;

Raspberry Sauce

Servings: 4 | Cooking Time: 10 Minutes

Ingredients:
- 1 cup fresh raspberries
- ¼ cup sugar
- 2 tablespoons water

Directions:
1. In a large saucepan over medium-high heat, cook the raspberries, sugar, and water, stirring frequently and mashing the raspberries with a spoon. Bring to a boil. Reduce the heat to low and simmer for 5 minutes.
2. Strain the sauce through a fine-mesh sieve to remove the seeds. Chill before serving.

Nutrition Info:
- Calories: 63; Total Fat: 0g; Saturated Fat: 0g; Carbohydrates: 16g; Fiber: 2g; Sodium: 1mg; Protein: <1g

Garlic Oil

Servings: 1 | Cooking Time: 5 Minutes

Ingredients:
- 1 cup olive oil
- 6 cloves garlic, sliced

Directions:
1. Heat the olive oil in a small saucepan over medium-low heat.
2. Add the garlic and cook at a low simmer, stirring often, for 5 minutes.
3. Strain the oil through a fine-meshed sieve and discard the solids.
4. Refrigerate the oil in a covered container for up to a week.

Nutrition Info:
- Calories: 108; Protein: 0g; Total Fat: 13g; Saturated Fat: 2g; Carbohydrates: 0g; Fiber: 0g; Sodium: 0mg;

Low-fodmap Mayonnaise

Servings: 1 | Cooking Time: 0 Minutes

Ingredients:
- 1 egg yolk
- 1 tablespoon red wine vinegar
- ½ teaspoon Dijon mustard
- ¼ teaspoon sea salt
- ¾ cup extra-virgin olive oil

Directions:
1. In a blender or food processor, combine the egg yolk, vinegar, mustard, and salt. Process for about 30 seconds until well combined. With a rubber spatula, scrape down the sides of the blender jar or food processor bowl.
2. Turn the blender or processor to medium speed. Very slowly, drip in the olive oil, 1 drop at a time as the processor or blender runs. After about 10 drops, leave the blender or processor running, then add the rest of the olive oil in a thin stream until it is incorporated and emulsified.
3. The mayo will keep refrigerated for up to 5 days.

Nutrition Info:
- Calories: 169; Total Fat: 20g; Saturated Fat: 3g; Carbohydrates: <1g; Fiber: 0g; Sodium: 63mg; Protein: <1g

Sweet Chili Garlic Sauce

Servings: 21 | Cooking Time: x

Ingredients:
- 1 pound fresh chili peppers, ends trimmed
- 1/16 teaspoon wheat-free asafetida powder
- 2 tablespoons safflower oil or other cooking oil
- ¼ cup rice wine vinegar
- ¼ cup brown sugar
- ¼ cup gluten-free fish sauce

Directions:
1. In a food processor add in chili peppers and asafetida powder. Process until minced.
2. In a medium sauté pan heat oil until shimmering on medium-high heat. Add in chili pepper mixture and cook 1 minute. Add in vinegar, sugar, and fish sauce and stir to combine. Turn heat to low and cook 25 minutes.
3. Before removing from heat taste sauce to see if you'd like it sweeter (add 1 tablespoon or more of brown sugar), saltier (add 1 tablespoon or more of fish sauce) or tangier (add 1 tablespoon or more of vinegar). Pour in an air-tight container or canning jar and store in pantry for 1 month or in refrigerator for up to 6 months.

Nutrition Info:
- Calories: 133, Fat: 6g, Protein: 2g, Sodium: 1,129mg, Carbohydrates: 19.

Olive Tapenade

Servings: 1 | Cooking Time: 0 Minutes

Ingredients:
- 1 cup chopped black olives
- 2 tablespoons Garlic Oil
- 2 tablespoons chopped fresh basil leaves
- 1 anchovy fillet, minced
- 1 tablespoon capers, chopped
- Juice of ½ lemon
- ½ teaspoon sea salt
- ⅛ teaspoon freshly ground black pepper

Directions:
1. In a small bowl, stir together all the ingredients until well mixed.

Nutrition Info:
- Calories: 61; Total Fat: 6g; Saturated Fat: <1g; Carbohydrates: 2g; Fiber: <1g; Sodium: 388mg; Protein: <1g

Autumn's Glaze

Servings:4 | Cooking Time:x

Ingredients:
- 2 tablespoons butter
- 1/4 cup hulled pumpkin seeds
- 1/8 teaspoon sea salt
- 3 tablespoons pure maple syrup, divided
- 1 tablespoon Dijon mustard

Directions:
1. Melt butter in a small saucepan and set aside.
2. Preheat broiler. Spread pumpkin seeds on a lined baking sheet. Drizzle 1 tablespoon of melted butter over pumpkin seeds. Sprinkle on salt. Toss seeds to coat. Broil for 1–2 minutes, or until seeds start to brown lightly. Remove from oven. Move seeds to serving dish and mix in 1 tablespoon maple syrup.
3. Return saucepan that contains the remaining tablespoon of butter to cooktop. Over medium heat, add remaining maple syrup and mustard. Bring just to a boil, then lower heat and simmer, uncovered, 1–2 minutes more to thicken.
4. The glaze and roasted seeds can be used to top any roasted poultry.

Nutrition Info:
- Calories: 140,Fat: 10g,Protein: 3g,Sodium: 120mg,Carbohydrates: 11.

Low-fodmap Vegetable Broth

Servings:8 | Cooking Time: 3 To 8 Hours

Ingredients:
- 3 carrots, roughly chopped
- 2 leeks, green parts only, roughly chopped
- 1 fennel bulb, roughly chopped
- 8 peppercorns
- 1 fresh rosemary sprig

Directions:
1. In a large stockpot or slow cooker, combine the carrots, leeks, fennel, peppercorns, and rosemary.
2. Fill the pot about ¾ full, with enough water to cover the ingredients.
3. If using a stockpot: Place the pot over medium-low heat and bring the liquid to a simmer.
4. Simmer for 3 hours.
5. If using a slow cooker: Cover the cooker, set the temperature to low, and cook for 8 hours.
6. Strain and discard the solids. Refrigerate or freeze the stock in 1-cup servings. The broth will keep in the refrigerator for about 5 days or in the freezer for up to 12 months.

Nutrition Info:
- Calories:15; Total Fat: 0g; Saturated Fat: 0g; Carbohydrates: 5g; Fiber: 0g; Sodium: 30mg; Protein: <1g

Basil Sauce

Servings:1 | Cooking Time:x

Ingredients:
- 1/4 cup tahini
- 1/4 cup fresh flat-leaf parsley leaves
- 1/4 cup coarsely chopped fresh chives
- 1 packed cup fresh basil
- Juice of 2 medium lemons
- 1/4 cup olive oil
- 1/4 teaspoon sea salt
- 1/4 teaspoon freshly ground black pepper

Directions:
1. Add all ingredients to a food processor. Blend until smooth. Store in an air-tight container in refrigerator for 5–7 days or in freezer for 3–4 months.

Nutrition Info:
- Calories: 56,Fat: 5g,Protein: 1g,Sodium: 42mg,Carbohydrates: 2.

Dill Dipping Sauce

Servings:3 | Cooking Time:x

Ingredients:
- 3 tablespoons chopped fresh dill
- 1 tablespoon lemon juice
- 7 ounces lactose-free sour cream
- 1/4 teaspoon salt

Directions:
1. In a food processor combine all ingredients and process until smooth. Use immediately or transfer to an airtight container and store in refrigerator for 3–4 days.

Nutrition Info:
- Calories: 64,Fat: 7g,Protein: 1g,Sodium: 125mg,Carbohydrates: 1.

Macadamia Spinach Pesto

Servings:1 | Cooking Time: 0 Minutes

Ingredients:
- 2 cups fresh baby spinach
- ½ cup fresh basil leaves
- ½ cup grated Parmesan cheese
- ¼ cup Garlic Oil
- ¼ cup macadamia nuts
- Zest of 1 lemon
- ½ teaspoon sea salt

Directions:
1. In a blender or food processor, combine all the ingredients.
2. Process until everything is well chopped and combined.

Nutrition Info:
- Calories:115; Total Fat: 12g; Saturated Fat: 2g; Carbohydrates: 1g; Fiber: <1g; Sodium: 189mg; Protein: 3g

Tangy Lemon Curd

Servings: 2 | Cooking Time: 10 Minutes

Ingredients:
- 1 cup granulated sugar
- 1 tablespoon finely grated lemon zest
- 1 cup lemon juice (from about 5 large lemons)
- 3 tablespoons chilled butter
- 3 eggs, lightly beaten

Directions:
1. In a medium saucepan over medium heat, whisk together the sugar, lemon zest, and lemon juice. Whisk in the butter and eggs, and cook the mixture, stirring constantly (be careful not to let it come to a boil), until it becomes thick, for 8 to 10 minutes.
2. Transfer the mixture to a ramekin or custard bowl, and cover with plastic wrap, pressing the plastic directly onto the surface of the curd to prevent a skin from forming, and chill for 4 hours.

Nutrition Info:
- Calories: 240; Protein: 3g; Total Fat: 12.4g; Saturated Fat: 7.2g; Carbohydrates: 32g; Fiber: 2g; Sodium: 42mg;

Maple Dressing

Servings: 3 | Cooking Time: x

Ingredients:
- 2 tablespoons pure maple syrup
- 2 tablespoons rice wine vinegar
- 2 tablespoons extra-virgin olive oil

Directions:
1. Combine all ingredients in a bowl or glass condiment jar and stir until completely combined. Store in an air-tight container at room temperature for 1–2 weeks.

Nutrition Info:
- Calories: 51, Fat: 5g, Protein: 0g, Sodium: 1mg, Carbohydrates: 3.

Caesar Salad Dressing

Servings: 11 | Cooking Time: x

Ingredients:
- 6 anchovy fillets packed in oil, drained and chopped
- 1/16 teaspoon wheat-free asafetida powder
- 2 large egg yolks
- 2 tablespoons fresh lemon juice
- 3/4 teaspoon Dijon mustard
- 2 tablespoons garlic-infused olive oil
- 1/2 cup extra virgin olive oil
- 3 tablespoons finely grated Parmesan cheese
- 1/4 teaspoon kosher salt
- 1 teaspoon freshly ground black pepper

Directions:
1. In a small bowl, mash anchovies and asafetida into a paste, then place in a medium bowl.
2. Whisk in egg yolks, lemon juice, and mustard. Slowly whisk in garlic-infused oil and then olive oil.
3. Whisk in Parmesan, salt, and pepper. Store in an air-tight container in refrigerator for 3–4 days.

Nutrition Info:
- Calories: 74, Fat: 7g, Protein: 3g, Sodium: 306mg, Carbohydrates: 1.

Aioli

Servings: 11 | Cooking Time: x

Ingredients:
- 1 teaspoon Dijon mustard
- 1 large egg
- 1/4 cup garlic-infused olive oil
- 3/4 cup olive oil
- 2 teaspoons freshly squeezed lemon juice
- 1/4 teaspoon kosher salt
- 1/8 teaspoon freshly ground black pepper

Directions:
1. Place mustard and egg in the bowl of a food processor fitted with a blade attachment.
2. With the motor running, slowly add garlic-infused oil followed by olive oil until completely combined, about 2 minutes.
3. Stop processor; add lemon juice, salt, and pepper and pulse until thoroughly mixed. If necessary, stop and scrape down the sides of the bowl using a rubber spatula to get any extra aioli, then continue to pulse until well combined.
4. Let aioli sit 30 minutes before using. If storing, place in a container with a tight-fitting lid in refrigerator up to 3 days.

Nutrition Info:
- Calories: 99, Fat: 11g, Protein: 0g, Sodium: 36mg, Carbohydrates: 0.

Artisanal Ketchup

Servings: 3 | Cooking Time: x

Ingredients:
- 3/4 cup Tomato Paste (see recipe in this chapter)
- 1 tablespoon white wine vinegar
- 1 tablespoon Simple Brown Syrup (see recipe in Chapter 16)
- 1/4 teaspoon dried oregano
- 1/8 teaspoon ground cumin
- 1/8 teaspoon ground cinnamon
- Water (as needed)

Directions:
1. Blend all ingredients in a food processor, adding water 1/4 cup at a time, until desired consistency is achieved.

Nutrition Info:
- Calories: 53, Fat: 2g, Protein: 1g, Sodium: 55mg, Carbohydrates: 8.

Basil "hollandaise" Sauce

Servings: 1 | Cooking Time: None

Ingredients:
- ½ cup cold rice milk
- ½ cup fresh basil leaves
- 4 teaspoons lemon juice
- 1 tablespoon nutritional yeast
- ½ teaspoon salt
- ⅛ teaspoon cayenne pepper
- ⅛ teaspoon turmeric
- ¼ teaspoon xanthan gum
- ½ cup light olive oil

Directions:
1. In a blender, combine the rice milk, basil, lemon juice, nutritional yeast, salt, cayenne, and turmeric, and process until smooth.
2. Add the xanthan gum and blend on high until the mixture becomes foamy.
3. With the blender running, slowly add the oil, blending until the sauce is thick.

Nutrition Info:
- Calories: 161; Protein: 1g; Total Fat: 17g; Saturated Fat: 2g; Carbohydrates: 3g; Fiber: 0g; Sodium: 203mg;

Low-fodmap Spicy Ketchup

Servings: 1 | Cooking Time: 20 Minutes

Ingredients:
- 2 tablespoons Garlic Oil (here)
- ¼ cup tomato paste
- ¼ cup light-brown sugar
- ½ teaspoon ground ginger
- ¼ teaspoon cayenne
- ¼ teaspoon ground allspice
- ⅛ teaspoon ground cinnamon
- ⅛ teaspoon ground cloves
- ¼ cup red-wine vinegar
- 1 (15-ounce) can tomato sauce
- ½ teaspoon salt
- ¼ teaspoon freshly ground black pepper

Directions:
1. Heat the Garlic Oil in a small saucepan over medium heat. Add the tomato paste and cook, stirring, for 1 minute.
2. Add the sugar, ginger, cayenne, allspice, cinnamon, and cloves, and cook, stirring frequently, until the sugar is fully dissolved. Stir in the vinegar, tomato sauce, salt, and pepper. Cook, stirring occasionally, for 15 to 20 minutes, until the sauce is very thick.
3. Let cool to room temperature. Serve immediately or store in a covered container in the refrigerator for up to a week.

Nutrition Info:
- Calories: 28; Protein: 1g; Total Fat: 0g; Saturated Fat: 0g; Carbohydrates: 7g; Fiber: 1g; Sodium: 289mg;

Homemade Mayonnaise

Servings: 1 | Cooking Time: None

Ingredients:
- 1 large pasteurized egg yolk
- 1½ teaspoons fresh lemon juice
- 1 teaspoon white wine vinegar
- ¼ teaspoon Dijon mustard
- ½ teaspoon salt
- ¾ cup light olive oil

Directions:
1. In a blender or food processor, combine the egg yolk, lemon juice, vinegar, mustard, and salt, and process to combine. With the processor running, slowly add the oil. Continue processing until all of the oil has been added and the mixture is thick.
2. Transfer to a storage container and store, covered, in the refrigerator for up to 3 days.

Nutrition Info:
- Calories: 113; Protein: 0g; Total Fat: 13g; Saturated Fat: 2g; Carbohydrates: 0g; Fiber: 0g; Sodium: 99mg;

Sweet Barbecue Sauce

Servings: 1 | Cooking Time: x

Ingredients:
- 1 cup Tomato Purée (see recipe in this chapter)
- 1 tablespoon Dijon mustard
- 1 tablespoon blackstrap molasses
- 1 1/2 tablespoons pure maple syrup
- 1/2 teaspoon ground cinnamon
- 1/2 teaspoon ground cumin
- 1/2 teaspoon dried oregano
- 1/2 teaspoon white wine vinegar
- 1/2 teaspoon arrowroot powder
- 1/2 teaspoon paprika
- 1/8 teaspoon ground red pepper
- 1/8 teaspoon nutmeg
- 1/8 teaspoon sea salt

Directions:
1. Bring all ingredients just to a boil in a small saucepan over medium-high heat. Lower heat and simmer, uncovered, 5–10 minutes, or until sauce thickens.

Nutrition Info:
- Calories: 25, Fat: 0g, Protein: 1g, Sodium: 100mg, Carbohydrates: 6.

Steakhouse Rub
Servings: 4 | Cooking Time: x

Ingredients:
- 1 teaspoon sea salt
- 1/4 teaspoon freshly ground black pepper
- 1/4 teaspoon ground mustard
- 1/2 teaspoon dried thyme
- 1/2 teaspoon dried rosemary, crumbled
- 1/4 teaspoon maple sugar
- 1/2 teaspoon orange zest

Directions:
1. Combine all ingredients in a small bowl.

Nutrition Info:
- Calories: 2, Fat: 0g, Protein: 0g, Sodium: 590mg, Carbohydrates: 0.

Strawberry Chia Seed Jam
Servings: 1 | Cooking Time: x

Ingredients:
- 1/2 pint (or 6 ounces) fresh strawberries
- 1 tablespoon lemon juice
- 2 1/2 tablespoons pure maple syrup
- 1 tablespoon chia seeds

Directions:
1. Add fruit, lemon juice, and maple syrup to a small saucepan and cook over medium-high heat. Cover. Stir occasionally until fruit begins to thicken, about 10 minutes.
2. Uncover and bring mixture to a boil until it develops a sauce-like consistency, about 5 minutes.
3. Stir in chia seeds and cook 2 more minutes. Stir again and then remove from heat.
4. Transfer jam to an airtight jar or other container and allow to cool, or refrigerate 2–3 hours before use. The jam will continue to thicken. Can be stored in refrigerator 2 weeks or frozen up to 2 months.

Nutrition Info:
- Calories: 26, Fat: 0g, Protein: 0g, Sodium: 2mg, Carbohydrates: 6.

Chimichurri Sauce
Servings: 1 | Cooking Time: None

Ingredients:
- 1 cup fresh flat-leaf parsley
- 1/4 cup lemon juice
- 1/4 cup olive oil
- 1/4 cup Garlic Oil (here)
- 1/4 cup fresh cilantro
- 3/4 teaspoon red-pepper flakes
- 1/2 teaspoon ground cumin
- 1/2 teaspoon salt

Directions:
1. Combine all the ingredients in a blender or food processor and process until smooth.
2. Use immediately or cover and refrigerate for up to a week.

Nutrition Info:
- Calories: 88; Protein: 1g; Total Fat: 9g; Saturated Fat: 1g; Carbohydrates: 3g; Fiber: 1g; Sodium: 203mg;

Italian Basil Vinaigrette
Servings: 5 | Cooking Time: 0 Minutes

Ingredients:
- 2 tablespoons apple cider vinegar
- 2 tablespoons extra-virgin olive oil
- 2 tablespoons Garlic Oil
- 2 tablespoons chopped fresh basil leaves
- 1/2 teaspoon Dijon mustard
- 1/4 teaspoon sea salt
- 1/8 teaspoon freshly ground black pepper

Directions:
1. In a small bowl, whisk together all the ingredients.
2. Whisk again just before serving.

Nutrition Info:
- Calories: 124; Total Fat: 14g; Saturated Fat: 2g; Carbohydrates: <1g; Fiber: 0g; Sodium: 118mg; Protein: <1g

Salsa Verde
Servings: x
Cooking Time: x

Ingredients:
- 2 handfuls of flat-leaf parsley, rinsed and dried
- 3 anchovy fillets in oil, drained (optional)
- 2 teaspoons capers, rinsed and drained
- 1 tablespoon garlic-infused olive oil
- 2 tablespoons olive oil
- 2 tablespoons fresh lemon juice, or to taste
- Salt and freshly ground black pepper

Directions:
1. Combine the parsley, anchovy fillets (if using), and capers in a food processor or blender and process until well combined.
2. Gradually add the garlic-infused oil and olive oil until well blended.
3. Add the lemon juice and salt and pepper to taste.
4. Spoon into a bowl or jar, cover, and store in the fridge for up to 5 days.

Nutrition Info:
- 53 calories; 1 g protein; 5 g total fat; 1 g saturated fat; 1 g carbohydrates; 0 g fiber; 158 mg sodium

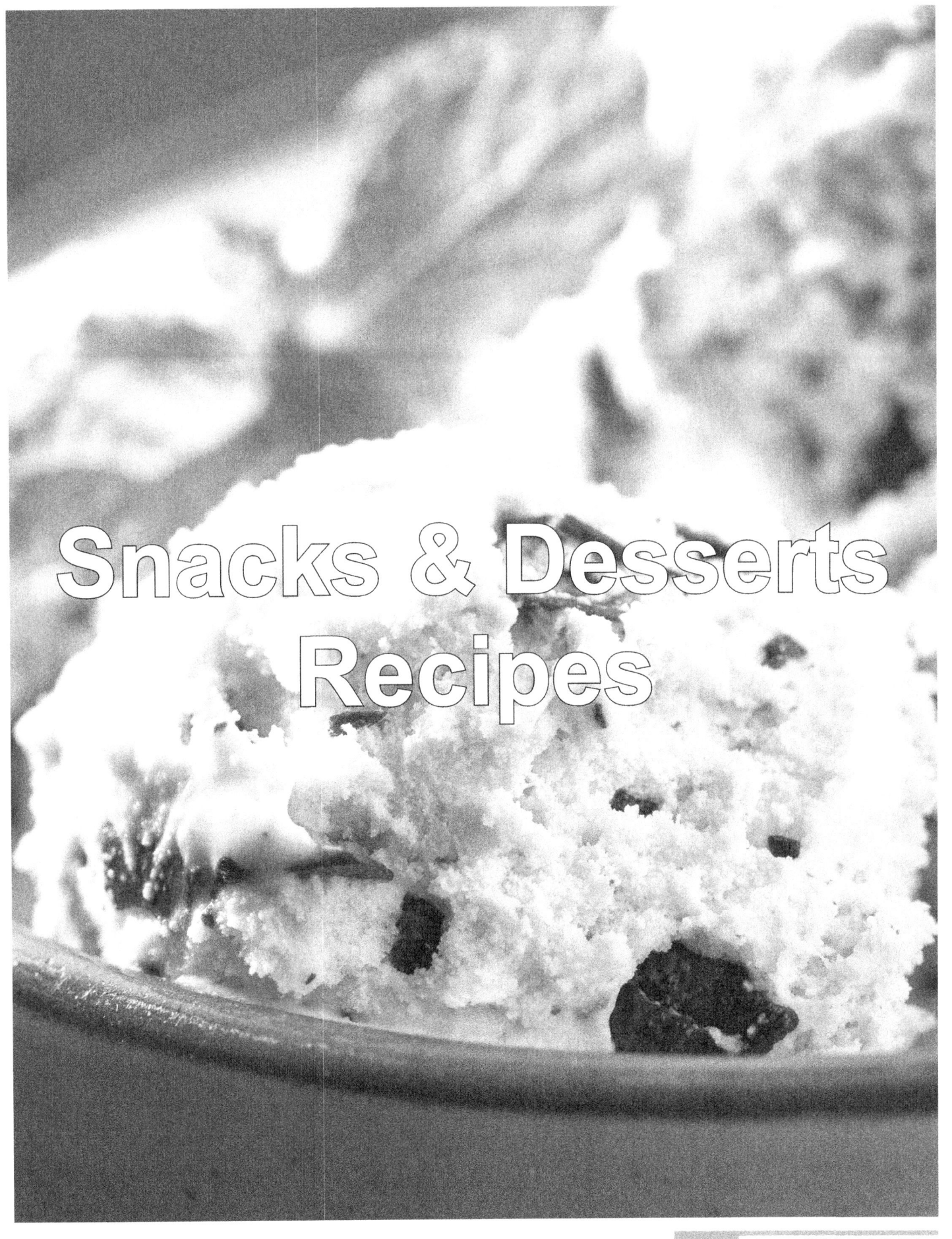

Snacks & Desserts Recipes

Snacks & Desserts Recipes

Cinnamon And Chestnut Flan

Servings:10 | Cooking Time:x

Ingredients:
- Nonstick cooking spray
- 1 batch Tart Crust dough, chilled
- ¾ cup (165 g) superfine sugar
- 2 tablespoons ground cinnamon
- One 14-ounce (396 g) can fat-free sweetened condensed milk
- One 8-ounce (225 g) package mascarpone or reduced-fat cream cheese, at room temperature
- 1½ cups (225 g) chestnut meal
- 4 large eggs
- Confectioners' sugar, for dusting
- Gluten-free, lactose-free ice cream, for serving

Directions:
1. Preheat the oven to 350°F (170°C). Grease a 9-inch (23 cm) fluted quiche pan with cooking spray.
2. Place the chilled dough between two sheets of parchment paper and roll out to a thickness of about ⅛ inch (2 to 3 mm). Ease the crust into the flan dish and trim the edges to neaten.
3. Line the crust with parchment paper, fill with pie weights or rice, and bake for 10 minutes, or until lightly golden. Remove from the oven and reduce the oven temperature to 325°F (160°C). Remove the weights and parchment.
4. Meanwhile, to make the filling, combine the superfine sugar, cinnamon, condensed milk, mascarpone, chestnut meal, and eggs in a food processor or blender and blend until smooth and well combined. Pour the filling into the warm crust.
5. Bake for 50 to 60 minutes, until set. Remove and let cool completely in the pan before serving.
6. Dust with confectioners' sugar and serve with ice cream.

Nutrition Info:
- 506 calories; 8 g protein; 21 g total fat; 7 g saturated fat; 71 g carbohydrates; 3 g fiber; 188 mg sodium

Easy Trail Mix

Servings:4 | Cooking Time: 0 Minutes

Ingredients:
- 1 cup dried bananas
- ½ cup raw unsalted almonds
- ¼ cup raw unsalted peanuts
- ¼ cup dried cranberries

Directions:
1. In a small bowl, mix all the ingredients.
2. Store in a resealable bag at room temperature for up to 1 month.

Nutrition Info:
- Calories:158; Total Fat: 11g; Saturated Fat: 1g; Carbohydrates: 13g; Fiber: 4g; Sodium: 2mg; Protein: 5g

Caramelized Upside-down Banana Cake

Servings:8 | Cooking Time: 25 Minutes

Ingredients:
- Butter or coconut oil for preparing the pan
- 2 tablespoons unsalted butter
- 2 tablespoons brown sugar
- 2 bananas, 1 sliced and 1 mashed, divided
- 2 eggs, lightly beaten
- ⅓ cup maple syrup
- ¼ cup unsweetened coconut milk
- 1 teaspoon vanilla extract
- ½ teaspoon baking soda
- 1 teaspoon distilled vinegar
- ⅓ cup coconut flour

Directions:
1. Preheat the oven to 350°F.
2. Grease a 9-inch cake pan with butter or coconut oil. Put the butter in the cake pan and place the pan in the oven for a few minutes while it is preheating. Once the butter is melted, remove the pan from the oven and tilt it around so that the butter thoroughly coats the bottom of the pan. Sprinkle the brown sugar over the melted butter and arrange the banana slices in the pan on top of the butter and sugar.
3. In a large bowl, combine the eggs, maple syrup, coconut milk, vanilla, baking soda, vinegar, and mashed banana, and mix well. Add the coconut flour, and stir to mix and eliminate any clumps.
4. Pour the batter on top of the banana slices in the pan and spread into an even layer.
5. Bake in the preheated oven until the top of the cake is lightly browned and the cake is set in the center, for about 25 minutes. Remove from the oven and cool completely in the pan on a wire rack.
6. Slide a butter knife around the edge of the cake to loosen it from the pan, then invert the cake onto a serving platter. Serve at room temperature.

Nutrition Info:
- Calories: 173; Protein: 3g; Total Fat: 7g; Saturated Fat: 5g; Carbohydrates: 26g; Fiber: 3g; Sodium: 130mg;

Parmesan Potato Wedges

Servings:4 | Cooking Time: 25 Minutes

Ingredients:
- 4 red potatoes, cut into wedges
- 2 tablespoons Garlic Oil
- ¼ cup grated Parmesan cheese
- ½ teaspoon sea salt
- ¼ teaspoon freshly ground black pepper

Directions:
1. Preheat the oven to 425°F.
2. In a small bowl, combine the potatoes, garlic oil, Parmesan cheese, salt, and pepper and toss to coat the potatoes with the cheese and oil. Spread the potatoes in a single layer on a rimmed baking sheet.
3. Bake for about 25 minutes, or until the potatoes are tender.

Nutrition Info:
- Calories:232; Total Fat: 9g; Saturated Fat: 2g; Carbohydrates: 34g; Fiber: 4g; Sodium: 313mg; Protein: 6g

Lemon Coconut Cupcakes

Servings:12 | Cooking Time: 25 Minutes

Ingredients:
- Cupcakes
- 1 ½ cups gluten-free, all-purpose flour
- ½ tsp xanthan gum
- 2 tsp of baking powder
- Pinch of salt
- 1 tbsp lemon zest
- ½ cup butter, room temperature
- ½ cup white sugar
- ½ cup brown sugar
- 2 eggs
- 1 tsp vanilla extract
- 2 ½ tbsp lemon juice
- ½ cup coconut yogurt
- Lemon butter icing
- ¾ cup butter
- 1 ½ cups powdered sugar
- 1 ½ tbsp lemon juice

Directions:
1. Preheat the oven to 350°F and grease a 12-muffin tin.
2. For the cupcakes, mix together the dry ingredients and put to the side.
3. In a large bowl, mix the butter and sugar until combined, then whisk together the eggs and vanilla until smooth before adding the lemon juice and blending. Add the dry ingredients and yogurt, alternating between them, beginning and ending with the dry ingredients. Mix well.
4. Spoon into muffin cups, filling ⅔ of the way. Place into the center of the oven and bake for 25 minutes. The tops should be golden. When a skewer or toothpick is inserted into them, it should come out clean. Leave to cool.
5. The icing is optional. To make the icing, mix room temperature butter and powdered sugar together with lemon juice until smooth. Then, use a knife to cover the top of the cupcakes after they have cooled.

Nutrition Info:
- 366g Calories, 17.5g Total fat, 4.4g Saturated fat, 49.4g Carbohydrates, 0.4 g Fiber, 2.7g Protein, 34.3g Sodium.

Crispy Gluten-free Chocolate Chip Cookies

Servings:24 | Cooking Time: 10 Minutes

Ingredients:
- 1 cup plus 2 tablespoons gluten-free flour (low-FODMAP blend such as King Arthur's)
- ½ teaspoon gluten-free baking powder
- ½ teaspoon gluten-free baking soda
- ½ teaspoon salt
- ½ cup butter, at room temperature
- ¼ cup sugar
- ½ cup packed light brown sugar
- 1 teaspoon vanilla extract
- 1 egg
- 1 cup semisweet chocolate chips

Directions:
1. Preheat the oven to 350°F.
2. Line a large baking sheet with parchment paper.
3. In a medium bowl, combine the flour, baking powder, baking soda, and salt.
4. In a large bowl using an electric mixer or in the bowl of a stand mixer, cream the butter and sugars together, mixing on medium speed, until well combined.
5. Add the egg and vanilla and beat to incorporate. Add the flour mixture in 2 additions, beating to incorporate after each addition. Stir in the chocolate chips.
6. Drop the cookies onto the prepared baking sheet by rounded spoonfuls, leaving at least 2 inches of space between them (you will need to bake in two batches or use two baking sheets).
7. Bake in the preheated oven for 10 minutes. Let the cookies cool on the baking sheet for 3 or 4 minutes before transferring them to a wire rack to cool completely.

Nutrition Info:
- Calories: 126; Protein: 1g; Total Fat: 7g; Saturated Fat: 4g; Carbohydrates: 16g; Fiber: 1g; Sodium: 112mg;

Sweet And Savory Popcorn

Servings: 7 | Cooking Time: 5 Minutes

Ingredients:
- ½ cup vegetable oil
- 1 cup popcorn kernels
- ⅓ cup brown sugar
- ⅓ cup white sugar
- 2 tsp salt, or to taste

Directions:
1. Blend together cranberries, butter, Greek yogurt, milk, banana, and chia seeds.
2. Add ice until the desired consistency is achieved.

Nutrition Info:
- 258g Calories, 16g Total fat, 2.2g Saturated fat, 24.8g Carbohydrates, 6.2 g Fiber, 3.7g Protein, 23.2g Sodium.

Berry Crumble

Servings: 3 | Cooking Time: 20 Minutes

Ingredients:
- Filling
- 1 cup blueberries, fresh or frozen
- 2 tbsp water
- 1 cup strawberries, fresh or frozen
- 1 ½ tsp white sugar
- 1 tbsp cornstarch, corn-based
- Crumble
- 1 cup gluten-free cornflakes
- ¼ cup packed brown sugar
- ¼ cup gluten-free flour
- 3 tbsp dried coconut, shredded
- 2 tbsp pumpkin seeds
- 4 tbsp butter, softened

Directions:
1. Preheat the oven to 350°F.
2. In a bowl, crush the cornflakes into small bits and mix them with the brown sugar, flour, coconut, and pumpkin seeds. Use the softened butter to work the dry mix into small crumbs, making sure there are no large lumps.
3. In an ovenproof dish, place the strawberries and blueberries, cutting the strawberries into smaller pieces if necessary. Over the berries, sprinkle the white sugar and cornstarch. Spread the crumble over the top evenly. Place the dish on a flat baking tray and cook in the oven for 20 minutes. The topping should be golden brown.
4. It is best served hot.

Nutrition Info:
- 425g Calories, 22.2g Total fat, 5.7g Saturated fat, 52.2g Carbohydrates, 3.6 g Fiber, 5.7g Protein, 22.6g Sodium.

Peanut Butter Cookies

Servings: 24 | Cooking Time: 10 Minutes

Ingredients:
- 1 cup sugar-free natural peanut butter
- ½ cup packed brown sugar
- 1 egg, beaten
- 1 teaspoon baking soda
- ½ teaspoon vanilla extract
- Pinch sea salt

Directions:
1. Preheat the oven to 350°F.
2. Line a baking sheet with parchment paper and set it aside.
3. In a medium bowl, mix the peanut butter and brown sugar.
4. Stir in the egg, baking soda, vanilla, and salt until well combined. Roll the dough into 24 teaspoon-size balls and place them on the prepared sheet. Flatten slightly with a fork in a crosshatch pattern.
5. Bake for about 10 minutes, or until the cookies puff and turn golden brown.

Nutrition Info:
- Calories: 78; Total Fat: 6g; Saturated Fat: 1g; Carbohydrates: 5g; Fiber: <1g; Sodium: 113mg; Protein: 3g

Maple-spiced Walnuts

Servings: 2 | Cooking Time: 8 Minutes

Ingredients:
- 2 tablespoons maple syrup
- 2 teaspoons olive oil
- 1 tablespoon water
- 2 cups walnut halves
- 1 tablespoon sugar
- 1 teaspoon coarse salt
- 1 teaspoon ground cumin
- ½ teaspoon ground coriander
- ⅛ teaspoon cayenne pepper

Directions:
1. Combine the maple syrup, oil, and water in a large skillet. Heat, stirring, over medium heat for about 5 minutes. Stir in the walnuts.
2. Add the sugar, salt, cumin, coriander, and cayenne pepper. Cook, tossing to coat the nuts well, for about 3 minutes more, until the nuts are lightly browned.
3. Transfer to a sheet of parchment paper, spread the nuts out into a single layer, separate them, and cool completely. Serve at room temperature.

Nutrition Info:
- Calories: 223; Protein: 8g; Total Fat: 20g; Saturated Fat: 1g; Carbohydrates: 8g; Fiber: 2g; Sodium: 242mg;

Rich White Chocolate Cake

Servings:12 | Cooking Time:x

Ingredients:
- Nonstick cooking spray
- 15 tablespoons (2 sticks minus 1 tablespoon/225 g) unsalted butter, cut into cubes
- 7 ounces (200 g) good-quality white chocolate, broken into pieces
- 2¼ cups (475 g) packed light brown sugar
- ¾ cup (65 g) soy flour
- ¾ cup (95 g) tapioca flour
- 1 cup (130 g) superfine white rice flour
- ½ cup (75 g) cornstarch
- 2 teaspoons xanthan gum or guar gum
- 1 teaspoon baking soda
- 1 teaspoon gluten-free baking powder
- 2 teaspoons vanilla extract
- 2 large eggs
- Confectioners' sugar, for dusting

Directions:
1. Preheat the oven to 300°F (150°C). Grease a 9-inch (23 cm) springform pan with cooking spray.
2. Combine the butter, white chocolate, brown sugar, and 1½ cups (375 ml) hot water in a medium heatproof bowl or the top part of a double boiler. Set over a saucepan of simmering water or the bottom part of the double boiler (make sure the bottom of the bowl does not touch the water) and stir until the chocolate and butter are melted and everything is well combined. Set aside to cool to room temperature.
3. Sift the soy flour, tapioca flour, rice flour, cornstarch, xanthan gum, baking soda, and baking powder three times into a medium bowl (or whisk in the bowl until well combined). Add the cooled white chocolate mixture, vanilla, and eggs and beat with a handheld electric mixer until smooth.
4. Pour the batter into the pan and bake for 45 minutes. Cover with foil and bake for 15 to 30 minutes more, until firm to the touch (a toothpick inserted into the center should come out clean).
5. Cool in the pan for 15 minutes, then remove the outer ring and turn out onto a wire rack to cool completely. Dust with confectioners' sugar before serving.

Nutrition Info:
- 496 calories; 7 g protein; 21 g total fat; 13 g saturated fat; 73 g carbohydrates; 1 g fiber; 196 mg sodium

Salted Caramel Pumpkin Seeds

Servings:16 | Cooking Time: 25 Minutes

Ingredients:
- Roasted seeds
- 2 cups pumpkin seeds
- 2 ½ tbsp sugar
- ¼ tsp cinnamon, ground
- ½ tsp ginger, ground
- Pinch of nutmeg
- 2 tsp water
- Salted caramel sauce
- 1 ½ tbsp butter
- 1 tbsp white sugar
- 1 ½ tbsp brown sugar
- ½ tsp rock salt

Directions:
1. Preheat the oven to 300°F.
2. Mix the pumpkin seeds, spices, and sugar with water. The seeds should be damp to allow the spices and sugar to stick.
3. Line a tray with parchment paper and grease it. Spread the seeds evenly over the tray, then bake in the oven for 25 minutes. The seeds should be golden and crunchy. Remember to mix the seeds up halfway through cooking.
4. When the seeds finish baking, place a saucepan over medium heat and melt the butter. Mix the sugar and salt into the butter, then cook for 2 minutes until the mixture is a deep golden color. Lower the heat. Mix the seeds into the caramel, transfer back to the tray, and let cool.

Nutrition Info:
- 124g Calories, 9.8g Total fat, 1.7g Saturated fat, 5.7g Carbohydrates, 1.1 g Fiber, 5.4g Protein, 4g Sodium.

Strawberry Ice Cream

Servings:4 | Cooking Time: -

Ingredients:
- 2 small bananas, firm and frozen
- 7 oz strawberries, frozen
- 5 tbsp coconut yogurt
- 2 tbsp maple syrup
- 1 tsp vanilla extract

Directions:
1. Chop the frozen fruit into small pieces, then place the ingredients into a food processor. Blend until smooth, making sure to scrape down the sides.
2. Taste the mixture and add maple syrup or vanilla extract as desired. Serve soft or freeze for a few hours before serving. Serve with chocolate fudge sauce.

Nutrition Info:
- 177g Calories, 4g Total fat, 3.5g Saturated fat, 37g Carbohydrates, 2.7 g Fiber, 1.2g Protein, 28.4g Sodium.

Herbed Rice Fritters With Parmesan Cheese

Servings:4 | Cooking Time: 16 Minutes

Ingredients:
- 2 cups cooked brown rice
- ½ cup freshly grated Parmesan cheese
- 1 tablespoon chopped fresh oregano
- ½ teaspoon salt
- ¼ teaspoon freshly ground black pepper
- 1 egg, lightly beaten
- ½ cup gluten-free all-purpose flour
- ¼ cup olive oil
- Finely chopped fresh parsley

Directions:
1. In a medium bowl, stir together the rice, Parmesan cheese, oregano, salt, pepper, and egg.
2. With slightly wet hands, form the mixture into eight cakes, about 2 inches in diameter. Place the cakes on a plate, cover with plastic wrap, and refrigerate for 30 minutes.
3. Place the flour on a plate and coat the chilled cakes in it.
4. Heat the olive oil in a large skillet over medium-high heat and cook the cakes, 4 at a time, until golden brown, for about 4 minutes per side. Garnish with the parsley and serve immediately.

Nutrition Info:
- Calories: 458; Protein: 15g; Total Fat: 22g; Saturated Fat: 7g; Carbohydrates: 53g; Fiber: 3g; Sodium: 574mg;

Chocolate Peanut Butter Cups

Servings:8 | Cooking Time: None

Ingredients:
- 1 cup all-natural creamy peanut butter
- 2 tablespoons coconut oil
- 2 tablespoons maple syrup
- Pinch salt
- 1 cup gluten-free, dairy-free, dark chocolate chips

Directions:
1. In a food processor, combine the peanut butter, coconut oil, maple syrup, and salt, and process until smooth and well combined. Spoon the mixture into cups of a mini muffin tin, dividing equally.
2. In the top of a double boiler set over simmering water, or in a microwave, melt the chocolate chips. Pour the melted chocolate over the peanut butter mixture in the muffin cups. Freeze for at least 30 minutes.
3. Pop the cups out of the muffin tin, using the tip of a sharp knife. Keep frozen until serving time, letting the cups sit at room temperature for 5 minutes before serving.

Nutrition Info:
- Calories: 312; Protein: 10g; Total Fat: 23g; Saturated Fat: 8g; Carbohydrates: 19g; Fiber: 2g; Sodium: 140mg;

Pineapple Salsa

Servings:2 | Cooking Time: None

Ingredients:
- 2 cups chopped pineapple
- 2 jalapeño chiles, seeded and finely chopped
- ¼ cup finely chopped cilantro
- ½ teaspoon salt
- Juice of 1 lime
- 1 tablespoon olive oil

Directions:
1. In a medium bowl, stir all of the ingredients together until well combined.
2. Let sit at room temperature for 15 to 20 minutes before serving to allow the flavors to blend.

Nutrition Info:
- Calories: 73; Protein: 1g; Total Fat: 4g; Saturated Fat: 1g; Carbohydrates: 11g; Fiber: 1g; Sodium: 292mg;

Fluffy Pancakes

Servings:16 | Cooking Time: 15 Minutes

Ingredients:
- Batter
- 1 ¼ cups gluten-free flour
- 3 tsp baking powder
- 2 tbsp white sugar
- ¾ cup lactose-free or coconut milk
- 1 egg
- ¾ tsp vanilla extract
- 2 tsp butter
- Serve
- ½ cup regular fat cream, whipped
- 8 tbsp strawberry jam

Directions:
1. In a bowl, whisk the dry ingredients and create a well in the middle. Add the milk, egg, and vanilla extract. Mix together until there are almost no lumps.
2. Test the batter. This is done by lifting the whisk out of the bowl. The batter should drizzle thickly back into the bowl; if it is too thick, add a tablespoon of milk.
3. Over medium heat, melt the butter in a non-stick pan. Wipe the pan with a paper towel to remove excess butter.
4. Place 2 tablespoons of batter per pancake into the pan. When bubbles appear on the top of the pancakes, flip them carefully and cook the other side until golden. Serve hot.

Nutrition Info:
- 116g Calories, 3.8g Total fat, 2g Saturated fat, 18.7g Carbohydrates, 0.2 g Fiber, 1.4g Protein, 9.4g Sodium.

Lemon Tartlets

Servings:x | Cooking Time:x

Ingredients:
- MAKES 12
- Nonstick cooking spray
- ½ cup (75 g) cornstarch
- 1¼ cups (300 ml) water
- Grated zest of 2 lemons
- ¾ cup (180 ml) fresh lemon juice
- 4 tablespoons (½ stick/60 g) unsalted butter, cut into cubes, at room temperature
- ⅔ cup (150 g) sugar
- 2 large egg yolks
- 1 batch Tart Crust dough, chilled
- Gluten-free, lactose-free ice cream, for serving

Directions:
1. Preheat the oven to 325°F (170°C). Grease twelve tartlet pans or a 12-cup muffin pan with cooking spray.
2. To make the filling, blend the cornstarch with 1 tablespoon of the water in a small saucepan to form a smooth paste. Add the remaining water, stirring to ensure there are no lumps, then add the lemon zest, lemon juice, butter, and sugar and stir over medium-low heat until thickened, 3 to 5 minutes. Remove from the heat and let cool for 10 minutes. Stir in the egg yolks. Pour into a bowl, cover, and refrigerate until cold.
3. Meanwhile, place the chilled dough between two sheets of parchment paper and roll out to a thickness of about ⅛ inch (2 to 3 mm). Cut out 12 rounds with a pastry cutter to fit the pan or cups. Place in the pan or cups and trim the edges to neaten. Bake for 12 to 15 minutes, until golden. Let cool on a wire rack.
4. Spoon the chilled lemon filling into the tartlet crusts and serve with ice cream.

Nutrition Info:
- 297 calories; 4 g protein; 15 g total fat; 9 g saturated fat; 39 g carbohydrates; 1 g fiber; 12 mg sodium

Dark Chocolate–macadamia Nut Brownies

Servings:18 | Cooking Time:x

Ingredients:
- Nonstick cooking spray
- 10 tablespoons (1¼ sticks/150 g) unsalted butter, cut into cubes
- 10½ ounces (300 g) good-quality dark chocolate, broken into pieces
- 1¼ cups (275 g) packed light brown sugar
- ⅔ cup (85 g) superfine white rice flour
- ¼ cup (35 g) cornstarch
- 1 teaspoon xanthan gum or guar gum
- 3 large eggs
- 2 teaspoons vanilla extract
- ½ cup (95 g) dark chocolate chips
- ½ cup (125 ml) light cream
- ¾ cup (100 g) roughly chopped macadamia nuts (optional)

Directions:
1. Preheat the oven to 325°F (160°C). Grease an 11 x 7-inch (29 × 19 cm) baking pan with cooking spray and line with parchment paper.
2. Combine the butter and chocolate in a medium saucepan over low heat and stir until melted and smooth. Add the brown sugar and stir until dissolved. Transfer to a large bowl and let cool to room temperature.
3. Sift the rice flour, cornstarch, and xanthan gum three times into a separate bowl (or whisk in a bowl until well combined).
4. Stir the eggs into the chocolate mixture, one at a time. Add the sifted flour mixture, vanilla, chocolate chips, cream, and macadamia nuts (if using). Mix well, spoon into the baking pan, and smooth the surface.
5. Bake for 20 minutes, then cover with foil and bake for 20 to 25 minutes more, until just firm to the touch.
6. Remove from the oven and let cool in the pan to room temperature. Transfer to the refrigerator for 2 to 3 hours or overnight, until firm.
7. Turn out onto a cutting board, peel off the parchment paper, and cut into squares to serve.

Nutrition Info:
- 278 calories; 3 g protein; 18 g total fat; 9 g saturated fat; 31 g carbohydrates; 2 g fiber; 23 mg sodium

Baked Oat Cup

Servings:12 | Cooking Time: 25 Minutes

Ingredients:
- 2 eggs
- 2 tbsp vegetable oil
- ½ cup water
- 1 cup lactose-free milk
- 2 tsp vanilla extract
- ⅓ cup brown sugar
- 2 ½ cups oats
- 2 tsp of baking powder
- 1 tsp cinnamon, ground
- Toppings: sliced strawberries and almonds, cranberries and walnuts, dark chocolate chips or shavings

Directions:
1. Preheat the oven to 350°F.
2. Line a muffin tin with paper liners.
3. Whisk the eggs, milk, and oil together in a bowl. Stir in the vanilla, sugar, oats, baking powder, and cinnamon. Leave the batter to thicken for a few minutes before stirring again.
4. Pour the batter evenly into muffin tin cups. Do not fill completely.
5. Add toppings then bake for 25 minutes.

Nutrition Info:
- 206g Calories, 6g Total fat, 1.4g Saturated fat, 31.5g Car-

bohydrates, 3.6 g Fiber, 6.5g Protein, 9g Sodium.

Rhubarb Custard Cup

Servings:4 | Cooking Time: 20 Minutes

Ingredients:
- Rhubarb
- 1 ¼ cups rhubarb, fresh
- 2 ½ tbsp raspberries, fresh or frozen
- Custard
- 4 tbsp custard powder, without milk or whey powder
- 4 cups lactose-free milk
- 1 ½ tbsp white sugar
- 1 tsp vanilla extract
- Layer
- Low-FODMAP muesli or crumble

Directions:
1. Weigh and chop the rhubarb. Place the rhubarb and raspberries into a saucepan, cover with warm water, and place over medium heat and bring to a simmer. Allow to simmer for 10 minutes, then drain the liquid using a sieve. Mash the fruit in the saucepan.
2. In a microwave bowl, mix together the custard powder, milk, and white sugar. Cook on high for 2 minutes and stir, repeating until thick. Add vanilla extract if the flavor is not sweet enough.
3. Layer the rhubarb, custard, and muesli/crumble into cups.

Nutrition Info:
- 431g Calories, 13.8g Total fat, 3.4g Saturated fat, 70.7g Carbohydrates, 5 g Fiber, 4.9g Protein, 26.1g Sodium.

Chocolate Lava Cakes

Servings:4 | Cooking Time: 15 Minutes

Ingredients:
- 4 tablespoons unsalted butter, plus more for preparing the ramekins
- 5 ounces dark chocolate, chopped
- 2 eggs
- 2 egg yolks
- ¼ cup granulated sugar
- ½ teaspoon vanilla extract
- 3 tablespoons gluten-free all-purpose flour
- ⅛ teaspoon xanthan gum
- 1 tablespoon unsweetened cocoa powder
- ⅛ teaspoon salt
- Powdered sugar, whipped cream, or Whipped Coconut Cream (here) for serving (optional)

Directions:
1. Preheat the oven to 425°F.
2. Butter the insides of 4 (4-ounce) oven-safe ramekins and place the ramekins in a baking dish.
3. In the top of a double boiler set over simmering water, combine the chocolate and 4 tablespoons butter, stirring frequently, until melted.
4. In a large bowl, whisk together the eggs, egg yolks, sugar, and vanilla until the mixture becomes thick and very pale yellow. While whisking, slowly add the melted chocolate-butter mixture to the egg mixture until well combined.
5. Stir in the flour, xanthan gum, cocoa powder, and salt. Transfer the mixture to the prepared ramekins in the baking dish, dividing equally.
6. Place the baking dish in the preheated oven and add water to the baking dish so that it comes halfway up the sides of the ramekins. Bake for about 15 minutes, until the centers of the cakes are just barely set.
7. Carefully remove the ramekins from the baking dish and transfer them to a wire rack. Cool for about 10 minutes. Before serving, run a butter knife around the edge of each cake to loosen it from the ramekin and then invert it onto a serving plate. Serve immediately, with a dusting of powdered sugar or a dollop of whipped cream or Whipped Coconut Cream.

Nutrition Info:
- Calories: 415; Protein: 7g; Total Fat: 27g; Saturated Fat: 16g; Carbohydrates: 38g; Fiber: 2g; Sodium: 146mg;

Banana Birthday Cake With Lemon Icing

Servings:16 | Cooking Time: 55 Minutes

Ingredients:
- Cake
- ½ cup white sugar
- ½ cup brown sugar
- 1 cup butter, softened
- 3 eggs, large
- 2 tsp vanilla extract
- 4 bananas, firm, mashed
- 1 tsp chia seeds, can be substituted with 1 ½ tsp guar gum
- 1 tbsp boiling water
- 2 tsp of baking soda
- ½ cup lactose-free milk
- 3 cups gluten-free flour
- 2 tsp of baking powder
- Icing
- 1 ½ tbsp lemon juice
- 5 tbsp butter
- 1 ½ cups powdered sugar
- 1 tbsp lemon zest

Directions:
1. Preheat the oven to 350°F. Grease a 10-inch round tin and line it with parchment paper.
2. In a bowl, mix the softened butter and sugar with a hand mixer until smooth and fluffy.
3. Add the vanilla and the eggs, one at a time.
4. Mash the bananas until there are 2 cups worth. Zest and juice the lemon and place the zest to the side. Add the banana and juice to the wet mix.
5. Dissolve the chia seeds in 1 tbsp of boiling water. Stir

until the consistency is thick and then add to the wet mixture.
6. Heat the milk in the microwave for 30 seconds, then mix the baking soda into it. Fold into the wet mixture.
7. Sift together the flour and baking powder. Mix the dry ingredients into the wet mixture and stir until fully mixed. Pour into the cake tin and bake in the center of the oven for 45-60 minutes. When the cake turns golden, check the middle of the cake with a skewer to see if it is cooked. Remove it from the oven and allow to cool.
8. For the icing, pour the powdered sugar into a bowl. Soften the butter, but do not melt it. Add the dairy into the bowl. Begin mixing and add the lemon juice. Mix until smooth.
9. Ice the cake once it is cool and top with the lemon zest.

Nutrition Info:
- 405g Calories, 18g Total fat, 2.8g Saturated fat, 56.8g Carbohydrates, 1.1 g Fiber, 3.7g Protein, 31g Sodium.

Lemon Tart

Servings:8 | Cooking Time:x

Ingredients:
- Nonstick cooking spray
- 1 cup (130 g) superfine white rice flour
- ½ cup (75 g) cornstarch, plus more for kneading
- ½ cup (45 g) soy flour
- 1 teaspoon xanthan gum or guar gum
- ¼ cup (55 g) superfine sugar
- 10 tablespoons (1¼ sticks/150 g) cold unsalted butter, diced
- About ½ cup (100 to 125 ml) ice water
- ¾ cup (165 g) superfine sugar
- One 8-ounce (225 g) package mascarpone (1 cup)
- 1 heaping tablespoon finely grated lemon zest
- ⅔ cup (165 ml) fresh lemon juice
- 4 large eggs
- Confectioners' sugar, for dusting

Directions:
1. Preheat the oven to 350°F (180°C). Grease a 9-inch (23 cm) fluted tart pan with cooking spray.
2. To make the crust, sift the rice flour, cornstarch, soy flour, and xanthan gum into a bowl. Transfer to a food processor, add the superfine sugar and butter, and process until the mixture resembles fine bread crumbs. While the motor is running, add the ice water (a tablespoon at a time) to form a soft dough.
3. Lightly sprinkle your work surface with cornstarch. Turn out the dough onto the work surface and knead until smooth. Wrap in plastic wrap and refrigerate for 30 minutes.
4. Place the dough between two sheets of parchment paper and roll out to a thickness of about ⅛ inch (2 to 3 mm). Ease the crust into the pan and trim the edges to neaten.
5. Line the crust with parchment paper, fill with pie weights or rice, and bake for 10 minutes, or until lightly golden. Remove the weights and parchment. Reduce the oven temperature to 325°F (160°C).
6. To make the filling, combine the superfine sugar, mascarpone, lemon zest, and lemon juice in a medium bowl and beat with a handheld electric mixer. Add the eggs one at a time, beating well between additions. Pour the filling into the warm crust and bake for 30 to 35 minutes, until set.
7. Cool completely in the pan. Dust with confectioners' sugar before serving.

Nutrition Info:
- 408 calories; 8 g protein; 24 g total fat; 8 g saturated fat; 42 g carbohydrates; 1 g fiber; 50 mg sodium

Amaretti

Servings:x | Cooking Time:x

Ingredients:
- MAKES 20–25
- 1 cup (120 g) almond flour (preferably finely ground)
- ¾ cup (120 g) confectioners' sugar
- 1 tablespoon plus 1 teaspoon cornstarch
- 2 large egg whites
- ⅓ cup (75 g) superfine sugar
- 1 teaspoon almond extract

Directions:
1. Preheat the oven to 325°F (170°C). Line two baking sheets with parchment paper.
2. Place the almond flour, confectioners' sugar, and cornstarch in a medium bowl and mix together well.
3. Beat the egg whites in a clean medium bowl with a handheld electric mixer until soft peaks form. Add the superfine sugar, 1 tablespoon at a time, and beat until shiny and stiff peaks form. Add the almond extract and beat to combine well. Gently fold in the almond flour mixture with a large metal spoon until just blended.
4. Place rounded teaspoons of the batter on the baking sheets, leaving room for spreading. Smooth the top of each cookie with the back of a metal spoon. Bake for 18 to 25 minutes, until lightly golden. Turn off the oven, leave the door ajar, and let the cookies cool and dry out in the oven.

Nutrition Info:
- 53 calories; 1 g protein; 2 g total fat; 0 g saturated fat; 8 g carbohydrates; 0 g fiber; 6 mg sodium

Chia Pudding

Servings:3 | Cooking Time: -

Ingredients:
- ¼ cup chia seeds
- 1 tbsp cocoa powder
- 1 tbsp peanut butter
- 1 tbsp maple syrup
- 1 can coconut milk

Directions:
1. Fill an airtight jar with all the ingredients.
2. Close the jar and shake, then remove the top and stir the

ingredients. Ensure that the bottom of the jar is clear. Shake again and place in the fridge for a minimum of 4 hours.
Nutrition Info:
• 386g Calories, 10g Total fat, 1g Saturated fat, 73g Carbohydrates, 20 g Fiber, 6g Protein, 24g Sodium.

Pineapple Sorbet
Servings:6 | Cooking Time: None
Ingredients:
- 1 small pineapple, peeled, cored, and cut into chunks
- 2 tablespoons lemon juice
- 1 cup sugar

Directions:
1. In a food processor, combine the pineapple and lemon juice, and process to a smooth purée. Add the sugar and process for another 1 to 2 minutes, until the sugar is completely dissolved.
2. Transfer the mixture to an ice cream maker and freeze according to the manufacturer's instructions.
3. Transfer to a freezer-safe container and freeze for several hours until very firm. Serve frozen.

Nutrition Info:
• Calories: 181; Protein: 1g; Total Fat: 0g; Saturated Fat: 0g; Carbohydrates: 48g; Fiber: 2g; Sodium: 2mg;

Vietnamese Shrimp-and-herb Spring Rolls
Servings:4 | Cooking Time: 50 Minutes
Ingredients:
- FOR THE DIPPING SAUCE
- ¼ cup rice vinegar
- ¼ cup fish sauce
- 1 cup water
- 1 tablespoon sugar
- FOR THE SPRING ROLLS
- 16 round rice-paper wrappers
- 1 cup fresh mint leaves
- 8 ounces cooked shrimp, peeled and halved lengthwise
- 2 cups cooked and cooled thin rice noodles
- 16 small lettuce leaves
- 3 cups bean sprouts
- 1 cup cilantro leaves

Directions:
1. To make the sauce, combine the vinegar, fish sauce, water, and sugar in a small saucepan set over medium heat. Cook, stirring, until the sugar is fully dissolved, for about 5 minutes. Remove from the heat and let cool completely.
2. Fill a wide, shallow bowl with warm water. Dunk 2 rice papers at a time into the water and let sit for about 1 minute, until softened. Lift the rice papers out of the water carefully and lay them, one on top of the other, on a clean dish towel.
3. Lay about 4 mint leaves in a line at the bottom of the rice paper, then add 4 shrimp halves on top of the mint. Top with a small handful of the rice noodles, a lettuce leaf, a small handful of bean sprouts, and a few cilantro leaves.
4. Fold the sides over the filling, then roll the rice paper up like a burrito and set on a serving platter, seam-side down.
5. Repeat with the remaining ingredients until you have 8 rolls. Halve the rolls and serve immediately, along with the dipping sauce.

Nutrition Info:
• Calories: 450; Protein: 25g; Total Fat: 4g; Saturated Fat: 0g; Carbohydrates: 62g; Fiber: 4g; Sodium: 1577mg;

Peanut Butter And Sesame Cookies
Servings:x | Cooking Time:x
Ingredients:
- MAKES 20–25
- 2 tablespoons (30 g) unsalted butter, at room temperature
- 1 cup (280 g) creamy peanut butter
- ¼ cup (55 g) packed light brown sugar
- 2 heaping tablespoons superfine sugar
- 2 large eggs, lightly beaten
- 1 teaspoon vanilla extract
- ¼ cup (35 g) sesame seeds
- ⅔ cup (85 g) superfine white rice flour
- ¾ cup (110 g) cornstarch
- ½ cup (45 g) soy flour
- ½ teaspoon baking soda
- 1 teaspoon xanthan gum or guar gum

Directions:
1. Preheat the oven to 350°F (170°C). Line two baking sheets with parchment paper.
2. Place the butter, peanut butter, brown sugar, and superfine sugar in a medium bowl and beat with a handheld electric mixer until creamy. Add the eggs, vanilla, and sesame seeds and beat well.
3. Sift the rice flour, cornstarch, soy flour, baking soda, and xanthan gum three times into a large bowl (or whisk in the bowl until well combined). Add to the peanut butter mixture and mix with a large metal spoon until well combined.
4. Shape the dough into walnut-size balls and place on the sheets, leaving a little room for spreading. Gently flatten to about ¼ inch (5 mm) thick.
5. Bake for 10 to 12 minutes, until golden.
6. Cool on the sheets for 5 minutes, then transfer to a wire rack to cool completely.

Nutrition Info:
• 130 calories; 5 g protein; 7 g total fat; 2 g saturated fat; 13 g carbohydrates; 1 g fiber; 84 mg sodium

Herbed Polenta "fries"
Servings:16 | Cooking Time: 40 Minutes
Ingredients:

- Olive oil for brushing
- 3¼ cups cold water
- 1 cup polenta
- 1 teaspoon chopped fresh sage
- 1 teaspoon chopped fresh rosemary
- ¾ teaspoon salt
- ½ cup grated Parmesan
- 2 tablespoons unsalted butter, cut into chunks

Directions:
1. Brush an 8-by-8-inch baking dish with olive oil.
2. In a medium saucepan set over medium heat, whisk together the water, polenta, sage, rosemary, and salt and bring to a boil. Reduce the heat to medium-low and cook, stirring continuously, until the mixture thickens, for 15 to 20 minutes. Add the cheese and butter, and stir to incorporate.
3. Spoon the polenta mixture into the prepared baking dish and spread it into a flat, even layer. Refrigerate, uncovered, for about 45 minutes, until set.
4. Preheat the broiler to high and line a large baking sheet with oiled aluminum foil.
5. Invert the pan of polenta to unmold it, then cut the polenta into sticks about 4 inches by 1 inch by 1 inch. Brush the sticks with oil and arrange them in a single layer on the prepared baking sheet. Broil for 15 to 20 minutes, until golden brown and crisp. Serve immediately.
6. Olives have a deep, rich umami flavor—especially helpful in seasoning when you can't use onions and garlic in your cooking.
7. This flavorful paste is fantastic spread on gluten-free crackers or cucumber rounds.
8. Dollop it in stew or soup to increase depth of flavor.
9. You won't taste any fishiness from the anchovies here, but feel free to omit them if you are vegetarian or they are simply not your cup of tea.
10. 1 cup pitted, cured black or green olives.
11. ¼ cup chopped flat-leaf parsley.
12. 1 tablespoon chopped fresh oregano.
13. 1 tablespoon capers, drained.
14. ½ teaspoon Dijon mustard.
15. 1 to 3 anchovy fillets (optional).
16. 1 tablespoon lemon juice.
17. 1½ teaspoons Garlic Oil (here).
18. 1½ teaspoons olive oil.
19. In a blender or food processor, combine all of the ingredients and pulse to a chunky paste.
20. You can also use a mortar and pestle to achieve the desired consistency.
21. Serve immediately or refrigerate for up to a week.

Nutrition Info:
- Calories: 314; Protein: 14g; Total Fat: 16g; Saturated Fat: 10g; Carbohydrates: 31g; Fiber: 1g; Sodium: 656mg;

Chocolate Peanut Butter Energy Bites
Servings:10 | Cooking Time: 2 Minutes

Ingredients:
- ½ cup smooth peanut butter
- 1 cup oats
- ⅓ cup maple syrup
- ¼ cup peanuts, roasted, chopped
- ¼ cup dark chocolate, 55%, finely chopped
- Pinch of salt

Directions:
1. In a bowl, mix the ingredients.
2. Once mixed, roll the mixture into balls (approximately 1 tablespoon in size, add more if there is mixture left once 10 balls have been rolled). They will need to be compressed as they are rolled. Store in an airtight container.

Nutrition Info:
- 240g Calories, 11g Total fat, 1g Saturated fat, 29g Carbohydrates, 4 g Fiber, 8g Protein, 9g Sodium.

No-bake Coconut Cookie Bars
Servings:12 | Cooking Time: None

Ingredients:
- 2 cups shredded unsweetened coconut
- ½ cup maple syrup
- ¼ cup coconut oil
- 1 teaspoon vanilla extract
- ¼ teaspoon salt

Directions:
1. Combine all of the ingredients in a food processor and process to combine well.
2. Transfer the mixture to a baking dish or rectangular cake pan (8-by-11-inch or similar capacity), and chill in the refrigerator for 1 hour.
3. Cut into 12 bars and serve chilled.

Nutrition Info:
- Calories: 122; Protein: 1g; Total Fat: 9g; Saturated Fat: 8g; Carbohydrates: 11g; Fiber: 1g; Sodium: 54mg;

Caramel Nut Bars
Servings:18 | Cooking Time:x

Ingredients:
- Nonstick cooking spray
- ½ cup (65 g) superfine white rice flour
- ¼ cup (45 g) potato flour
- ⅓ cup (50 g) cornstarch
- ¼ cup (55 g) superfine sugar
- ¼ teaspoon baking soda
- ¼ teaspoon gluten-free baking powder
- 1 teaspoon xanthan gum or guar gum
- 4 tablespoons (½ stick/60 g) unsalted butter, cut into cubes, at room temperature
- 1 large egg, beaten
- 1 teaspoon vanilla extract
- 1 cup (220 g) packed light brown sugar
- 10 tablespoons (1 stick plus 2 tablespoons/150 g) unsalted butter, cut into cubes, at room temperature

- ⅓ cup (80 ml) light cream
- 3 tablespoons plus 1 teaspoon cornstarch
- ½ cup (65 g) roasted unsalted pecans, roughly chopped
- ⅔ cup (110 g) roasted unsalted Brazil nuts (skin on), roughly chopped
- ½ cup (70 g) roasted unsalted macadamia nuts, halved

Directions:
1. Preheat the oven to 350°F (180°C). Grease an 11 x 7-inch (28 x 18 cm) baking pan with cooking spray and line with parchment paper, leaving an overhang on the two long sides to help lift out the bars later.
2. Sift the rice flour, potato flour, cornstarch, superfine sugar, baking soda, baking powder, and xanthan gum together three times into a bowl (or whisk in the bowl until well combined). Rub in the butter with your fingertips. Add the egg and vanilla and mix with a large metal spoon until well combined. As the mixture becomes more solid, use your hands to bring it together to form a ball.
3. Roll out the dough between two sheets of parchment paper to a thickness of ¼ inch (5 mm). Gently fit into the bottom of the pan and prick all over with a fork. Refrigerate for 10 minutes.
4. Bake for 10 to 12 minutes, until the crust is firm and lightly golden. Set aside to cool, but leave the oven on.
5. To make the topping, combine the brown sugar and butter in a large saucepan over medium heat and stir until the butter has melted and the mixture comes to a boil. Remove from the heat and stir in the cream and cornstarch, mixing until smooth. Add the pecans, Brazil nuts, and macadamia nuts. Return the pan to medium heat and stir until the mixture comes to a boil. Reduce the heat to low and cook gently for 2 to 3 minutes more, until the mixture is thick and sticky.
6. Spread the nut topping evenly over the crust and bake for 15 minutes, or until the topping is bubbling. Let cool completely in the pan, then transfer to a board, remove the parchment paper, and cut into small (or large!) pieces to serve.

Nutrition Info:
- 278 calories; 3 g protein; 20 g total fat; 8 g saturated fat; 25 g carbohydrates; 1 g fiber; 39 mg sodium

Chocolate-mint Bars

Servings:18 | Cooking Time:x

Ingredients:
- Nonstick cooking spray
- 8 tablespoons (1 stick/120 g) unsalted butter, cut into cubes, at room temperature
- ⅓ cup (75 g) superfine sugar
- ½ cup (65 g) superfine white rice flour
- ¼ cup (20 g) soy flour
- ½ cup (75 g) cornstarch
- 1 teaspoon xanthan gum or guar gum
- 2 heaping tablespoons unsweetened cocoa powder
- 1 cup (160 g) confectioners' sugar
- One 8-ounce (225 g) package reduced-fat cream cheese, at room temperature
- 3 to 4 teaspoons peppermint extract
- ½ cup plus 2 tablespoons (120 g) vegetable shortening, melted
- 4 ounces (115 g) good-quality dark chocolate, broken into pieces
- 1 tablespoon plus 1 teaspoon light cream
- 3 scant tablespoons (30 g) vegetable shortening

Directions:
1. Preheat the oven to 325°F (170°C). Grease an 11 x 7-inch (29 × 19 cm) baking pan with nonstick cooking spray and line with parchment paper.
2. Combine the butter and sugar in a medium bowl and beat with a handheld electric mixer until thick and pale.
3. Sift the rice flour, soy flour, cornstarch, xanthan gum, and cocoa three times into a separate bowl (or whisk in a bowl until well combined). Add to the creamed butter and sugar and stir with a large metal spoon until well combined. Gently gather into a ball and knead lightly in the bowl. Press the dough into the prepared pan.
4. Bake for 10 to 15 minutes, until lightly browned. Set aside to cool completely.
5. To make the peppermint filling, combine the confectioners' sugar, cream cheese, and peppermint extract in a bowl and beat with a handheld electric mixer until well combined. Add the shortening and beat for 1 to 2 minutes, until smooth. Spread the filling evenly over the cookie crust and refrigerate until set.
6. To make the chocolate topping, combine the dark chocolate, cream, and shortening in a small saucepan and stir over low heat until melted and well combined.
7. Remove the pan from the refrigerator and spread the chocolate topping over the peppermint filling. Refrigerate until set, then cut into squares to serve.

Nutrition Info:
- 247 calories; 2 g protein; 19 g total fat; 9 g saturated fat; 19 g carbohydrates; 1 g fiber; 42 mg sodium

Chocolate Truffles

Servings:25 | Cooking Time:x

Ingredients:
- 7 ounces (200 g) gluten-free vanilla cookies, finely crushed (about 2 cups)
- ⅓ cup (35 g) unsweetened cocoa powder
- ⅓ cup (80 ml) sweetened condensed milk
- 2 tablespoons rum or brandy (optional)
- 1½ cups (150 g) gluten-free chocolate sprinkles

Directions:
1. Mix together the crushed cookies and cocoa in a medium bowl. Add the condensed milk and rum (if using) and mix with your hands to form a firm dough.
2. Pour the chocolate sprinkles into a shallow bowl. Shape

teaspoons of the truffle mixture into balls with your hands. Toss in the chocolate sprinkles to coat. Refrigerate until firm.

Nutrition Info:
- 99 calories; 1 g protein; 2 g total fat; 0 g saturated fat; 20 g carbohydrates; 1 g fiber; 29 mg sodium

Brownie Cupcakes With Vanilla Icing
Servings:12 | Cooking Time: 20 Minutes

Ingredients:
- Cupcakes
- ½ cup butter
- 9 tbsp dark chocolate
- 2 eggs, large
- ¼ cup lactose-free milk
- 1 tsp vanilla extract
- 1 cup gluten-free flour
- 3 tbsp cocoa powder
- ¾ cup brown sugar
- ¼ tsp of baking powder
- ¾ tsp of baking soda
- Pinch of salt
- Icing
- ½ cup butter
- 1 ½ cups powdered sugar
- ½ tsp vanilla extract
- 2 drops food coloring of choice
- Edible cake decorating pearls, optional

Directions:
1. Preheat the oven to 350°F. Line a muffin tray with cupcake liners.
2. Chop the chocolate roughly and melt it in the microwave with the butter for 15 seconds at a time, stirring in between.
3. Whisk the eggs, milk, and vanilla extract together until smooth, then add in the melted butter and chocolate.
4. In a separate bowl, mix the dry ingredients together then add in the wet mixture. Mix until the batter is smooth. Spoon an even amount of mixture into each cupcake liner.
5. Bake for 15 minutes, then check with a skewer. The top of the cupcakes should look slightly cracked and the skewer should come out clean. Remove the cupcakes from the oven and let the tin cool for 5 minutes before placing the cupcakes onto a cooling rack.
6. To make the icing, soften the butter, but don't melt it. Mix the butter, powdered sugar, vanilla extract, and 2 drops of food coloring in a bowl until it is smooth and creamy. If it is too dry, add a small amount of water. Ice the cupcakes once they are cool and decorate.

Nutrition Info:
- 365g Calories, 19,9g Total fat, 4.7g Saturated fat, 43.9g Carbohydrates, 1.7 g Fiber, 3.2g Protein, 30.8g Sodium.

Citrus Rice Tart With Raspberry Sauce
Servings:8 | Cooking Time:x

Ingredients:
- Nonstick cooking spray
- 1 cup (200 g) medium-grain white rice
- ¼ cup (55 g) sugar
- ⅓ cup (50 g) cornstarch
- 3 large eggs
- ½ cup (150 ml) light cream
- ½ teaspoon vanilla extract
- Grated zest of 1 orange
- ¾ cup (180 ml) fresh orange juice
- Grated zest of 1 lemon
- One 15-ounce (425 g) can raspberries in syrup, drained, reserving the juice (see Note)
- ¼ cup (60 ml) raspberry juice (from the can)
- 1 heaping tablespoon confectioners' sugar

Directions:
1. Preheat the oven to 325°F (160°C). Grease a 9-inch (23 cm) fluted tart or pie pan with cooking spray.
2. Bring 6½ cups (1.5 liters) water to a boil in a large saucepan. Add the rice and sugar and cook, stirring occasionally, for 12 minutes, or until the rice is tender. Drain and rinse under cold water to cool.
3. Combine the cornstarch, eggs, cream, vanilla, orange zest and juice, and lemon zest in a medium bowl. Add the rice and mix well. Pour into the tart pan and bake for 35 to 40 minutes, until just set.
4. Remove from the oven and let cool to room temperature, then refrigerate for 2 to 3 hours.
5. Remove from the refrigerator 30 minutes before serving. If your pan has a removable bottom, slip off the outer rim.
6. To make the raspberry sauce, blend all the ingredients in a blender or food processor. Serve drizzled over the tart.

Nutrition Info:
- 234 calories; 4 g protein; 4 g total fat; 2 g saturated fat; 45 g carbohydrates; 1 g fiber; 37 mg sodium

RECIPES

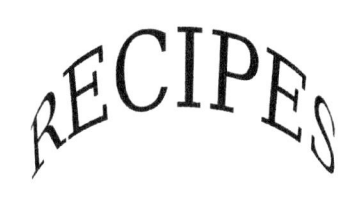

DATE

RECIPES	Salads	Meats	Soups
SERVES	Grains	Seafood	Snack
PREP TIME	Breads	Vegetables	Breakfast
COOK TIME	Appetizers	Desserts	Lunch
FROM THE KITCHEN OF	Main Dishes	Beverages	Dinners

INGREDIENTS

DIRECTIONS

NOTES

SERVING ☆☆☆☆☆

DIFFICULTY ☆☆☆☆☆

OVERALL ☆☆☆☆☆

Date: _____

MY SHOPPING LIST

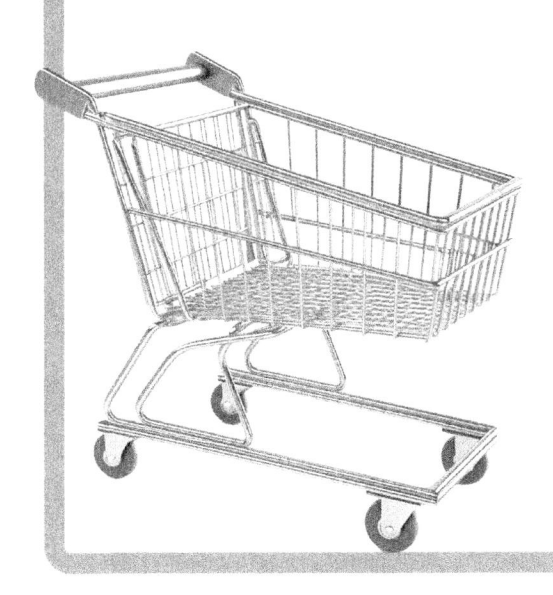

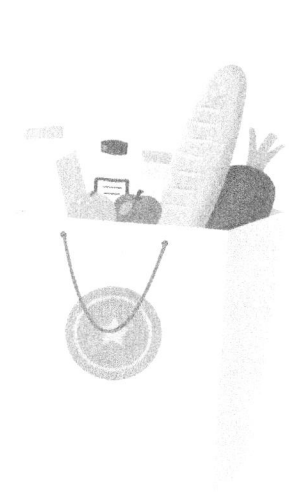

Appendix A: Measurement Conversions

BASIC KITCHEN CONVERSIONS & EQUIVALENTS

DRY MEASUREMENTS CONVERSION CHART

3 TEASPOONS = 1 TABLESPOON = 1/16 CUP

6 TEASPOONS = 2 TABLESPOONS = 1/8 CUP

12 TEASPOONS = 4 TABLESPOONS = 1/4 CUP

24 TEASPOONS = 8 TABLESPOONS = 1/2 CUP

36 TEASPOONS = 12 TABLESPOONS = 3/4 CUP

48 TEASPOONS = 16 TABLESPOONS = 1 CUP

METRIC TO US COOKING CONVERSIONS

OVEN TEMPERATURES

120 °C = 250 °F

160 °C = 320 °F

180° C = 350 °F

205 °C = 400 °F

220 °C = 425 °F

LIQUID MEASUREMENTS CONVERSION CHART

8 FLUID OUNCES = 1 CUP = 1/2 PINT = 1/4 QUART

16 FLUID OUNCES = 2 CUPS = 1 PINT = 1/2 QUART

32 FLUID OUNCES = 4 CUPS = 2 PINTS = 1 QUART = 1/4 GALLON

128 FLUID OUNCES = 16 CUPS = 8 PINTS = 4 QUARTS = 1 GALLON

BAKING IN GRAMS

1 CUP FLOUR = 140 GRAMS

1 CUP SUGAR = 150 GRAMS

1 CUP POWDERED SUGAR = 160 GRAMS

1 CUP HEAVY CREAM = 235 GRAMS

VOLUME

1 MILLILITER = 1/5 TEASPOON

5 ML = 1 TEASPOON

15 ML = 1 TABLESPOON

240 ML = 1 CUP OR 8 FLUID OUNCES

1 LITER = 34 FL. OUNCES

WEIGHT

1 GRAM = .035 OUNCES

100 GRAMS = 3.5 OUNCES

500 GRAMS = 1.1 POUNDS

1 KILOGRAM = 35 OUNCES

US TO METRIC COOKING CONVERSIONS

1/5 TSP = 1 ML

1 TSP = 5 ML

1 TBSP = 15 ML

1 FL OUNCE = 30 ML

1 CUP = 237 ML

1 PINT (2 CUPS) = 473 ML

1 QUART (4 CUPS) = .95 LITER

1 GALLON (16 CUPS) = 3.8 LITERS

1 OZ = 28 GRAMS

1 POUND = 454 GRAMS

BUTTER

1 CUP BUTTER = 2 STICKS = 8 OUNCES = 230 GRAMS = 8 TABLESPOONS

WHAT DOES 1 CUP EQUAL

1 CUP = 8 FLUID OUNCES

1 CUP = 16 TABLESPOONS

1 CUP = 48 TEASPOONS

1 CUP = 1/2 PINT

1 CUP = 1/4 QUART

1 CUP = 1/16 GALLON

1 CUP = 240 ML

BAKING PAN CONVERSIONS

1 CUP ALL-PURPOSE FLOUR = 4.5 OZ

1 CUP ROLLED OATS = 3 OZ 1 LARGE EGG = 1.7 OZ

1 CUP BUTTER = 8 OZ 1 CUP MILK = 8 OZ

1 CUP HEAVY CREAM = 8.4 OZ

1 CUP GRANULATED SUGAR = 7.1 OZ

1 CUP PACKED BROWN SUGAR = 7.75 OZ

1 CUP VEGETABLE OIL = 7.7 OZ

1 CUP UNSIFTED POWDERED SUGAR = 4.4 OZ

BAKING PAN CONVERSIONS

9-INCH ROUND CAKE PAN = 12 CUPS

10-INCH TUBE PAN = 16 CUPS

11-INCH BUNDT PAN = 12 CUPS

9-INCH SPRINGFORM PAN = 10 CUPS

9 X 5 INCH LOAF PAN = 8 CUPS

9-INCH SQUARE PAN = 8 CUPS

Appendix B : Recipes Index

A

Abundantly Happy Kale Salad 31
Aioli 78
Amaranth Breakfast 20
Amaretti 89
Artisanal Ketchup 78
Asian-style Pork Meatballs 69
Atlantic Cod With Basil Walnut Sauce 37
Autumn's Glaze 77

B

Bacon And Zucchini Crustless Quiche 21
Bacon Mashed Potatoes 30
Baked Chicken And Mozzarella Croquettes 62
Baked Moroccan-style Halibut 42
Baked Oat Cup 87
Baked Tofu And Vegetables 56
Baked Tofu Báhn Mì Lettuce Wrap 54
Banana Birthday Cake With Lemon Icing 88
Banana Oatcakes 19
Banana Toast 19
Basic Baked Scallops 41
Basic Mayonnaise 74
Basil "hollandaise" Sauce 79
Basil Omelet With Smashed Tomato 18
Basil Sauce 77
Basil Vinaigrette Salad Dressing 16
Beef Stir-fry With Chinese Broccoli And Green Beans 70
Beetroot Dip 31
Berry Crumble 84
Blue Cheese And Arugula Salad With Red Wine Dressing 30
Blueberry Lime Smoothie 21
Blueberry, Lime, And Coconut Smoothie 17
Breakfast Ratatouille With Poached Eggs 22
Breakfast Tortillas 19
Brownie Cupcakes With Vanilla Icing 93
Butter Lettuce Salad With Poached Egg And Bacon 32

C

Caesar Salad Dressing 78
Caramel Nut Bars 91
Caramelized Squash Salad With Sun-dried Tomatoes And Basil 26
Caramelized Upside-down Banana Cake 82
Carrot Cake Porridge 22
Cedar Planked Salmon 42
Cheese Strata 48
Chia Pudding 89
Chia Seed Carrot Cake Pudding 17
Chicken And Dumplings Soup 27
Chicken And Rice With Peanut Sauce 66
Chicken Liver Pâté With Pepper And Sage 22
Chicken Parmigiana 64
Chicken Pockets 65
Chicken Tenders 63
Chili-cheese Muffins 23
Chili-rubbed Pork Chops With Raspberry Sauce 60
Chimichurri Chicken Drumsticks 66
Chimichurri Sauce 80
Chinese Chicken 61
Chipotle Tofu And Sweet Potato Tacos With Avocado Salsa 58
Chive Dip 29
Chocolate Lava Cakes 88
Chocolate Peanut Butter Cups 86
Chocolate Peanut Butter Energy Bites 91
Chocolate Truffles 92
Chocolate-mint Bars 92
Cinnamon And Chestnut Flan 82
Cinnamon Spice Granola 19
Citrus Rice Tart With Raspberry Sauce 93
Citrusy Swordfish Skewers 43
Classic Coleslaw 30
Coconut Cacao Hazelnut Smoothie Bowl 21
Coconut Rice 28
Coconut Shrimp 37
Coconut-crusted Fish With Pineapple Relish 43
Coconut-curry Tofu With Vegetables 50
Collard Green Wraps With Thai Peanut Dressing 51
Cornmeal-crusted Tilapia 38
Creamy Halibut 38
Creamy Seafood Soup 33
Creamy Smoked Salmon Pasta 61
Crêpes With Cheese Sauce 18

Crispy Baked Chicken With Gravy 67
Crispy Gluten-free Chocolate Chip Cookies 83
Crispy Noodle Cakes With Chili Sauce 20
Crunchy Granola 22
Cucumber Salad 15
Curried Squash Soup With Coconut Milk 49

D

Dark Chocolate–macadamia Nut Brownies 87
Dijon-roasted Pork Tenderloin 69
Dill Dipping Sauce 77
Dressed-up Eggs 15

E

Easy Breakfast Sausage 17
Easy Onion- And Garlic-free Chicken Stock 28
Easy Pan Chicken 68
Easy Trail Mix 82
Egg Wraps 20
Egg-free Caesar Dressing 75
Eggplant And Chickpea Curry 52

F

Fennel Pomegranate Salad 33
Feta Crab Cakes 44
Fiesta Salsa 75
Fish And Chips 45
Fish With Thai Red Curry Sauce 70
Fluffy Pancakes 86
Fried Eggs With Potato Hash 24

G

Garden Veggie Dip Burgers 63
Garlic Oil 76
Garlic-infused Oil 75
Ginger Sesame Salad Dressing 75
Ginger-berry Rice Milk Smoothie 16
Glazed Salmon 42
Green Dragon Smoothie Bowl 24
Grilled Chicken Parmigiana 60
Grilled Cod With Fresh Basil 40
Grilled Halibut With Lemony Pesto 41
Grilled Swordfish With Pineapple Salsa 43

H

Hearty Lamb Shank And Vegetable Soup 34
Herbed Polenta "fries" 91
Herbed Rice Fritters With Parmesan Cheese 86
High-fiber Muffins With Zucchini And Sunflower Seeds 21
Homemade Mayonnaise 79

I

Italian Basil Vinaigrette 80
Italian-herbed Chicken Meatballs In Broth 68

J

Jubilant Muesli Mix 15

K

Kale And Red Bell Pepper Salad 34
Kale Sesame Salad With Tamari-ginger Dressing 34
Kale-pesto Soba Noodles 49

L

Lamb And Vegetable Pilaf 65
Latin Quinoa-stuffed Peppers 57
Lemon And Mozzarella Polenta Pizza 53
Lemon Coconut Cupcakes 83
Lemon Tart 89
Lemon Tartlets 87
Lemon Thyme Chicken 62
Lemon-pepper Shrimp 71
Lemony Grilled Zucchini With Feta And Pine Nuts 26
Light Tuna Casserole 39
Low-fodmap Mayonnaise 76
Low-fodmap Poultry Broth Or Meat Broth 73
Low-fodmap Spicy Ketchup 79
Low-fodmap Vegetable Broth 77
Low-fodmap Worcestershire Sauce 74
Luscious Hot Fudge Sauce 73

M

Mac 'n' Cheeze   49
Macadamia Spinach Pesto   77
Maple Dressing   78
Maple-glazed Salmon   45
Maple-spiced Walnuts   84
Mediterranean Flaky Fish With Vegetables   40
Mediterranean Noodles   55
Melon And Yogurt Parfait   18
Mild Lamb Curry   60
Mixed Grains, Seeds, And Vegetable Bowl   55
Mom's Chicken Salad   35
Moroccan-spiced Lentil And Quinoa Stew   58
Mussels In Chili, Bacon, And Tomato Broth   28

N

No-bake Coconut Cookie Bars   91

O

Olive Tapenade   76
Orange-ginger Salmon   61
Orange-maple Glazed Carrots   28

P

Pan-fried Chicken With Brown Butter–sage Sauce   63
Parmesan Potato Wedges   83
Pasta With Pesto Sauce   54
Pasta With Tomato And Lentil Sauce   51
Pb&j Smoothie   17
Peanut Butter And Sesame Cookies   90
Peanut Butter Cookies   84
Pecan-crusted Maple-mustard Salmon   66
Pesto Ham Sandwich   34
Pesto Noodles   24
Philly Steak Sandwich   35
Pineapple Fried Rice   52
Pineapple Salsa   86
Pineapple Sorbet   90
Poached Salmon With Tarragon Sauce   42
Polenta With Roasted Vegetables And Spicy Tomato Sauce   50
Polenta-crusted Chicken   71
Pork And Fennel Meatballs   63
Potato Leek Soup   31
Prosciutto Di Parma Salad   30
Pumpkin Maple Glaze   73
Pumpkin Maple Roast Chicken   66

Q

Quick Meatloaf Patties   71
Quinoa Breakfast Bowl With Basil "hollandaise" Sauce   23
Quinoa Porridge   23
Quinoa With Cherry Tomatoes, Olives, And Radishes   29
Quinoa With Swiss Chard   32

R

Raspberry Sauce   76
Rhubarb Custard Cup   88
Rhubarb Ginger Granola Bowl   16
Rice Paper "spring Rolls" With Satay Sauce   26
Rich White Chocolate Cake   85
Rita's Linguine With Clam Sauce   37
Roast Vegetables   33
Roasted Potato Wedges   28
Roasted Squash And Chestnut Soup   26
Roasted Sweet Potato Salad With Spiced Lamb And Spinach   27
Roasted Vegetable Soup   32
Roasted-veggie Gyros With Tzatziki Sauce   48
Roman Egg Drop Soup   35

S

Salmon Cakes With Fresh Dill Sauce   40
Salmon Noodle Casserole   39
Salmon With Herbs   44
Salsa Verde   80
Salted Caramel Pumpkin Seeds   85
Savory Muffins   16
Scrambled Tofu   15
Seafood Risotto   40
Sesame Rice Noodles   29
Shrimp And Cheese Casserole   38
Shrimp Puttanesca With Linguine   38
Shrimp With Cherry Tomatoes   44
Snapper With Tropical Salsa   71
Sole Meunière   43
Soy-infused Roast Chicken   70
Spicy Pulled Pork   62

Spinach And Feta-stuffed Chicken Breast 67
Steakhouse Rub 80
Strawberry Chia Seed Jam 80
Strawberry Ice Cream 85
Strawberry Smoothie 17
Stuffed Peppers With Ground Turkey 69
Stuffed Rolled Roast Beef With Popovers And Gravy 64
Stuffed Zucchini Boats 48
Summer Vegetable Pasta 53
Summery Fish Stew 37
Sun-dried Tomato Pesto 75
Sweet And Savory Popcorn 84
Sweet Barbecue Sauce 79
Sweet Chili Garlic Sauce 76

T

Tahini Dressing 74
Tangy Lemon Curd 78
Tempeh Enchiladas With Red Chili Sauce 52
Tempeh Lettuce Wraps 55
Tempeh Tacos 47
Thai Red Curry Paste 74
Thai Sweet Chili Broiled Salmon 67
Tilapia Piccata 41
Tofu And Red Bell Pepper Quinoa 47
Tofu Burger Patties 57
Tomato Paste 73
Turkey Dijon 68
Turkey-ginger Soup 29
Turmeric Rice With Cranberries 55

V

Vegan Noodles With Gingered Coconut Sauce 47
Vegan Pad Thai 51
Vegan Potato Salad, Cypriot-style 56
Vegetable And Rice Noodle Bowl 54
Vegetable Fried Rice 56
Vegetable Stir-fry 51
Veggie Dip 31
Vietnamese Shrimp-and-herb Spring Rolls 90

W

Watercress Zucchini Soup 57

Z

Zucchini Pasta Alla Puttanesca 53
Zucchini Pizza Bites 50
Zucchini Ribbon Salad With Goat Cheese, Pine Nuts, And Pomegranate 32

Printed in Great Britain
by Amazon